Beyond Conception

The New Politics of Reproduction

Patricia Spallone

Bergin & Garvey Publishers, Inc.
Massachusetts

First published in 1989 in the United States of America by
BERGIN & GARVEY PUBLISHERS, INC.
670 Amherst Road, Granby, Mass. 01033.

Printed in Hong Kong

Library of Congress Cataloging-in-Publication Data
Spallone, Patricia.
   Beyond conception.
   Bibliography: p.
   1. Human reproductive technology—Moral
and ethical aspects.   2. Feminism.   I. Title.
RG133.5.S63   1989   176   88–7590
ISBN 0–89789–199–6
ISBN 0–89789–198–8

For Allison August

Contents

Acknowledgements

My mother and my father taught me to think and feel and have confidence. I am forever beholden to them.

This book like so many others comes out of a women's movement, and so I owe a debt of gratitude to countless numbers of women, some whose names I can think of, more of them nameless.

Jalna Hanmer rekindled my concern over the new reproductive technologies, and encouraged me to write this book. For her help and to all the women of the FINRRAGE network, special thanks and my deepest affections. Thanks to Maria Mies, Farida Akhter, Ramona Koval, Sultana Kamal, Cindy de Wit, Gena Corea and Lene Koch for their correspondence. Lene, my dear friend, deserves credit for the title *Beyond Conception*.

I am enormously grateful to many women in Britain with whom I have been working on these issues and who have generously given me so much of their time and creative energy and affection. Debbie Steinberg read more drafts of this book than she probably cares to remember; for her sustaining encouragement and perceptive criticisms, many many thanks. Marilyn Crawshaw has been a guiding light from the moment I met her. Deepest thanks to Christine Crowe and Sarah Franklin for reading drafts and their kindly, wise criticisms; and to Annette Burfoot, Renate Klein, Noe Mendelle, Kerry Perkins and Jalna Hanmer for many helpful discussions. I gained experience and knowledge working with women in the York and Leeds Women's Reproductive Rights Campaigns and especially wish to thank Penny Bainbridge, Dorothy Large, Veronica Ford, Marilyn Crawshaw, and Debbie Hughes in York. I am also grateful to the women at the Women's Reproductive Rights Information Centre in London; their constant efforts in providing up-to-date information on reproductive health and practices has helped many women, including me.

Women's Studies at the University of York supported me with their interest throughout this work. Sara Knowles, Susan Miller, Treva Broughton, Joanna de Groot and Anne Akeroyd helped in many ways. Delia Davin spent much time with me labouring over the very first paper I ever wrote as a Women's Studies student. I carried out much of the research and writing of this book while a Visiting Scholar in the Institute for Research in the Social Sciences from 1986–7, for which I appreciate the support of Mary Maynard and Keith Hartley. Thanks also to Jean Wall in Women's Studies, who made life easier by knowing where to go, who to see, and how to mould a photocopier to one's needs; and to Elizabeth Heaps and the library staff of the University who were most helpful.

To the biologists: for their loans of research materials, for helpful discussions and their careful listening, I warmly thank Peter Hogarth and Henry Leese at the University of York (England), Jerome Strauss at the University of Pennsylvania (US), and Francis Webb at the World Health Organisation in Geneva.

To Jo Campling and Steven Kennedy at Macmillan, my thanks for helpful and enjoyable discussions and correspondence. Jo helped me learn the ropes of writing for publication.

To my enduring friends Ada Bello, Allison August and Baruch Ticho, for sending me news clippings and articles from the USA, and to David White, who encouraged, aided and sustained me in this endeavour in all ways from the practical to the intangible, thank you and much love.

PATRICIA SPALLONE

Introduction

In the first week of July 1985, women from sixteen countries met in Vällinge, Sweden, at an emergency conference on new developments in reproductive and genetic technology. A resolution emerged to resist the development and application of these technologies globally, in the interests of all women, in the knowledge that these technologies are harmful to women, a destruction of women's physical integrity, an exploitation of women's procreativity, and yet another attempt to undermine women's struggle for control of our own reproduction. The group of over seventy women has grown to hundreds since then, continuing an international network of information sharing and feminist resistance. The name of the network became FINRRAGE, the Feminist International Network of Resistance to Reproductive and Genetic Engineering.

A few months earlier in Bonn, West Germany, a similar resolution was passed at the conference Women Against Gene Technology and Reproductive Technologies (19–21 April). Since then many more meetings have been held on the local, national and international levels, to move forward a critical feminist stance and a demand for a woman-centred approach to the issues. Gene and reproductive technologies are the wrong approach to the wrong questions. From the Bonn resolution:

> We consider it time for the backgrounds, sources of finance, entwinement of interests, also of so-called basic research, to be discussed by as many of those concerned as possible, and on a world scale. (*Frauen Gegen Gentechnik und Reproduktionstechnik*, 1985)

In this book I consider some of these backgrounds, *as part a of*

1

larger political process of women's learning, feminist analysis and awareness–making. Specifically, I have tried to break the silence of the laboratories, to bring into the foreground what is going on in the background. This book then is especially concerned with the accountability of scientists, medical scientists, including obstetricians and gynaecologists, to women.

I came to work on these issues from an interest in the women's health movement and reproductive rights movement, and from my experience working in chemistry and biochemistry for twelve years in research laboratories at the University of Pennsylvania School of Medicine in the USA. In 1984, I began researching the area of reproductive technologies while a student on the MA course in Women's Studies at the University of York, in England. As I explored the medical and scientific literature, ethical reports, and the report of the British Government Warnock Inquiry on *in vitro* fertilisation (IVF, the 'test-tube' baby procedure) and related issues, it became clear that the whole area of reproductive technology, and its correlative genetic engineering, were of great social and political importance for all people, especially women.

It became apparent that in the dominant 'public' debate over these issues, and in the less public debates among medical scientists themselves, women were being ignored as the subject on whom these technologies are implemented. Paradoxically, one message from medical scientists and the state is that these technologies present another reproductive 'choice'. Also, an undercurrent eugenic meaning was apparent, touted as a 'new' (better) eugenics. Clearly, the technologies were not invented to serve *women's* needs, but the various needs and desires of medical scientists, research scientists, and the state, to further technological 'progress' and to aid population control aims, all of which requires the use of women to those ends. Today, few advocates of the new reproductive technologies admit this basic precondition, at least publicly. There are some, however, who are blatantly clear about their advocacy of reproductive engineering, as we will see.

Much of this book is based on medical and scientific literature. Scientific papers and books are important modes of communication of the international scientific community, and the written word reflects the turning of scientific 'data' into scientific knowledge. The social meaning of reproductive and genetic technologies is in part constructed in the scientific discourse. I feel it is essential to examine the medical – scientific discourse on these issues to get a full picture of what is going on in the reproductive technology area. In industrial countries, scientific knowledge and technology impinge on our everyday lives. And Western science and technology has been and continues to be imposed on people in developing countries as part of development aid and population control programmes.

Looking back, I know that part of my interest in taking my original research on these issues further stems from my own working experience in 'medical' research laboratories. A great deal of the research, certainly all the projects I was involved with, were in the realm of so-called 'basic' research; these projects are not fundamentally medical projects. They are scientific explorations about biological events. I am aware of the changes that are taking place in laboratory research: the greater dependence on sophisticated instrumentation to gather scientific data; the greater emphasis now on molecular genetics; the greater prestige of those medical doctors who spend their time in laboratories doing what is considered 'basic' research as compared to doctors who spend their time attending to patients or carrying out epidemiological studies; the resurgence in the 1980s of an intimate relationship between scientists working in universities and in government laboratories with industrial and military interests; the absurdity of the 'scientific freedom' principle in the light of the politics of research science (who gets funding, why, etc.).

The most difficult hurdle for me was coming to terms with the criticism that if we resist IVF and 'human embryo' research, women with fertility problems will be denied a reproductive right and a reproductive choice. I hope to show that IVF is not about infertility, but rather is being applied to women in the name of infertility therapy.

Analogies usually are inadequate, but I would like to offer one that was impressed on me while writing this book. Over the years while working with hazardous chemicals in open rooms (inadequately protected by any measure of common sense and occupational safety standards), I have become 'sensitised', for want of a better word, to a variety of commonly used chemicals, to perfumes, and to other environmental contaminents. Actually, I experienced chemical poisoning and still suffer chemical poisoning reactions to toxins most people can 'live with'. I no longer enjoy choices others enjoy about my work, life-style or activities, nor easy health. This is a chronic pervasive imposition. It has made me reassess the concept 'choice', the power of concepts such as social 'normality', and especially with respect to IVF issues, a little of what it must mean to a woman with fertility problems *not* to have the choice to reproduce biologically. I know my experience forced me to reassess the activities of science, what disability means, choice and beyond, to an analysis of the way we in industrialised countries relate to our environment and to technology.

This book is a critique of technologies of reproduction. I do not mean to imply that removing the technologies will automatically give back to women control over our own bodies. Women can be subjugated within a society which constructs a completely non-technological reproductive practice. For example, Margaret Atwood's futuristic novel, *The Handmaid's Tale*, considers a society built on a literal reading of the Bible, but a society in which most women cannot reproduce biologically because their fertility has been affected by environmental pollution. There is no contraceptive technology, no conception technology, and no pregnancy intervention technology. Those women who can reproduce biologically are subjugated to a role of 'two-legged wombs', and all other women are subjugated to alternative roles as wives, servants, prostitutes, or Econowives (all-purpose women).

One of the main purposes of this book is to show how technology redefines the meaning of reproduction in society to the detriment of women, how technology sets a repressive ethic of reproduction, and in turn how repressive social relations provide the conditions for the technologies to happen.

I keep in mind an international perspective overall, but in particular look at the situation in Great Britain because (i) it was necessary to focus the critique in some way, especially because of the complexity of issues; (ii) the pioneering work of Robert Edwards and Patrick Steptoe in England prompted renewed interest and involvement of doctors and scientists all over the world to apply IVF and related procedures to women; (iii) the British Committee of Inquiry on IVF issues (the Warnock Committee), and their endorsement of the use of IVF/human embryo research on women prompted many other countries to follow suit; and (iv) I have been living in Britain and working and campaigning with women here on these issues.

I use the phrase 'Third World' but am not comfortable with the categorisation of such a diversity of geographies, histories, and cultures for the majority of the people in the world. Yet, as the economist Joyce Kolko puts it: 'One economic system girdles the globe and subjects all of these diverse states that possess subsistence-wage workers and raw materials to ruthless exploitation and violent repression. It is the impact of imperialism that permits such categorisation' (1974, p. 118).

At this point I wish to clarify my viewpoint. I speak often of the relationship between patriarchal social relations and the new reproductive technologies. As Maria Mies does, I take patriarchy to denote 'the historical and societal dimension of women's exploitation and oppression' (Mies, 1986, p. 37).

Mies continues, 'the concept *capitalism* is expressive of the contemporary manifestation, or the latest development of this system' (p. 38). Thus, one cannot fully appreciate the medical science approach to reproductive technology without understanding the emergence of the biotechnology industry. Indeed, IVF itself created a whole industry and markets. And as Annette Burfoot found in her study of the development of commercial interests in IVF, a management investment company in Australia, CP Ventures Ltd, chose IVF as one of the two highest profile areas for investment (Burfoot, 1987). IVF is developing in a big way because of these financial interests, and others. For example, Robert Edwards was privately funded by the Ford Foundation in the early years of his work on 'human IVF', when the Medical Research Council would not grant public funding for the projects. Of course, Edwards' apointment at Cambridge allowed him the use of public resources and facilities for this work. Although my analysis in this book does not directly address the commercial interests and funding which influence the development and practice of the new reproductive and genetic technologies, these must be understood as a crucial part of the motivation behind the technologies.

In Chapter 1, 'Setting the Ethic', I set the stage for the rest of the book by naming and placing the central issues and criticisms which will be developed further in following chapters. This chapter serves as an overview.

Chapter 2, 'The Status of the Embryo', looks closely at one of the most important terms of reference in the debate on reproductive and genetic technologies. Scientific knowledge and reproductive technologies are being used by 'experts' to construct a distinctive meaning of an embryo (fetus) which is repressive to women. The image of a disembodied embryo is historical. It still depends, as it has in the past, on the image of motherhood, not the realities of motherhood. But today, more and more, that image of the embryo is being constructed from technology-knowledge (what scientists 'know' about embryos). The concepts of *fetal* rights, *fetal* neglect, and the fetus-as-patient are eroding women's rights and interests, and our identity as whole human persons.

Chapter 3, 'IVF on Women', is a brief description of the IVF protocol, reclaiming women's identity as the subject of these procedures. It serves to show how inadequate is the facile term 'IVF'. This chapter also lays a foundation for following chapters.

Chapter 4, 'The Realm of Medicine', places IVF and related methods in their medical context. Here I discuss the medical meaning of infertility, why IVF does not address women's fertility problems in the interests of women, and how medical definitions of infertility-as-disease increase medical authority over women's lives.

Chapter 5, 'The Status of Scientific Knowledge', follows to show that women are the experimental subjects (objects) of 'pure' laboratory research into 'human reproduction'. I then look at the interrelationships between the pursuit of scientific knowledge about women's reproduction and the technologies of reproduction, and what it means for women. I consider this a key chapter, in that it shows how the construction of scientific knowledge about women's reproductive processes *requires* the exploitation of women's bodies as the raw materials of research. This, I believe, is one of the most important points this book has to make.

Chapters 6 and 7 on 'The New Genetics' and 'The New Eugenics' broaden my analysis on the status of scientific knowledge and its meaning for women. Here I look at the interrelationships between the natural sciences, especially genetics, and eugenics (the science of selective breeding to 'improve' the human stock). As I explored the intellectual history of eugenics and genetics/evolutionary theory, it became clear that women are perceived by scientist-eugenists as the raw materials of scientific 'progress' in reproduction (where 'progress' means scientists should 'guide' the evolution of the human species), that women's bodies are the primary site of the population planners, and that women are the human subjects who are most burdened with genetic technologies. I briefly place reproductive and genetic engineering within the scope of biotechnologies generally. These chapters serve to point out some historical connections and overlapping concerns.

Chapter 8, 'A Matter of State Interest', is about the role of government committees and laws in forging the social meaning of the new reproductive technologies. Here I look at the collusion of medical science 'experts' and agents of the state in undermining women's sexual and reproductive autonomy, and how the state would mould the meaning of reproductive technology in the interests of patriarchy.

Throughout these chapters I counter the new technologies with ways women have been responding to medical and social control of reproduction. The final chapter, 'Transforming Reality', offers some afterthoughts on the nature of reproductive/genetic technology and feminist proposals.

To aid the newcomer to these issues there is a glossary of technical terms for easy reference; more detailed descriptions appear within the text. The appendix, 'What's What', is a list of medical and scientific organisations in Great Britain which appear regularly throughout the book, again for easy reference while reading.

I have tried not to over-reference the material within the text, but as this book is aimed as a springboard for further research, I record sources where I felt it would be helpful. I quote IVF advocates liberally, to make clear exactly where they stand on these issues. The section, 'Published Sources', organises the material in the References and can be used for further reading.

I use inverted commas (quotation marks) around words or phrases in two ways. In one instance, inverted commas stress that the actual words were used by a speaker. For example I write, The American Fertility Society recommended that surrogacy be considered a 'clinical experiment'. This shows that they themselves used the phrase 'clinical experiment'. In a second instance, the inverted commas signal that a word does not adequately convey the reality from a woman-centred perspective. For example, I often write 'human reproduction' when a commentator is actually talking about experimentation on women's reproduction (women's fertility, pregnancy, birth). I am stressing two things, that a speaker is using those words or that concept, and that the usage is faulty from a women-centred perspective.

1

Setting the ethic

On 25 July 1978, in England, the world's first 'test-tube' baby, Louise Brown, was born to Lesley and John Brown. The birth marked the realisation by a research scientist, Robert Edwards, and his colleague, gynaecologist Patrick Steptoe, that fertilisation of a woman's egg and a man's sperm which took place outside the female body and in a laboratory dish could be placed back into the woman's body and develop to term. The first live birth from 'test tube' fertilisation, or what scientists call *in vitro* fertilisation or IVF, came after years of experimentation: experimentation which included removing eggs from women's bodies, growing the eggs under laboratory conditions, and eventually entailed inserting the fertilised eggs into women's wombs in the hope that pregnancy would result.

IVF, the procedure which first entails physiological manipulation of women's bodies to extract eggs, was an invention of the natural science, biology. IVF is one of many biological 'breakthroughs' of the second half of the twentieth century, along with genetic engineering. Biological science, like physics and chemistry before it, has come of age. We are in the midst of a revolution in biology, where control of human reproductive capacities are considered of great importance. In his 1968 book, *The Biological Time-Bomb*, Gordon Rattray Taylor discussed the IVF research then being conducted, the implications of 'pre-natal adoption' of embryos created by IVF, sex-choice, artificial wombs, and the future prospect of 'baby factories'. He discussed all these in the context of other scientific breakthroughs, such as organ transplantation, genetic engineering, and the creation of living viruses from

8

non-living molecules. It was a decade before the first 'test-tube' baby was born. Under a heading 'Biological Control' he wrote,

The radical nature of what is happening can perhaps best be conveyed by a comparison. We can now create, on a commercial scale by chemical processes, substances which previously we had to look for in nature, and even substances which never previously existed. Whereas before we had to make do with what nature provided, now we can decide what we want; this may be called chemical control. Similarly, in the coming century, we shall achieve biological control: the power to say how much life, of what sort, shall exist where. We shall even be able to create forms of life which never existed before. (p. 16)

So, the work aimed at creating 'test-tube' babies that scientists were conducting in the 1960s and 70s was controversial, even within the scientific community. In the early 1970s, an ethical debate accompanied the technical papers on IVF progress in US and British medical and scientific journals.[1] However, little was said about the effect of using these procedures on women. Rather, the in-house debate addressed broad, so-called humanistic concerns, concentrating on embryos and the effect on 'society', but leaving women invisible. The fact that women's bodies are needed to perform 'human IVF' experimentation was left unexamined. The fact that biological control of 'human reproductive capacities' means primarily the control of women's fertility and pregnancy was not acknowledged.

In 1973, the *Journal of Reproductive Medicine* reviewed this debate, in which scientists, philosophers, ethicists and theologians participated. For example, questions arose as to whether tampering with reproduction would be good for humanity or whether it gave scientists and doctors too much control over 'human reproduction' (Kass, 1971). Among those who were wary of the new direction biologists were taking in 'human reproduction' was James Watson, who co-discovered the molecular structure of DNA (the genetic material, what genes are made of), the discovery which turned the tide of biology in 1953. Due to the controversy over the new reproductive technologies, IVF research slowed down in the USA, resulting in a *de facto* ban on government funding for 'human IVF' research. As of 1987, all research on 'human IVF' in the USA is privately funded, at least formally.

Before 1978, the two prominent research groups carrying out 'human IVF' research were Edwards and Steptoe in England and the team of Carl Wood in Australia. Soon after the birth of Louise Brown, the international scientific community rallied, and by mid-1980 IVF clinics and research facilities existed in almost every country that takes part in the Western scientific establishment. Early doubts about the profound changes in human relations which the technology would inevitably bring subsided among members of the scientific community. The discussion in the medical and scientific literature revolved around clinical applications of IVF with respect to benefits, risks (mostly to the potential offspring, not to the woman), and the place of IVF in 'pure' scientific research. Less than a decade after the first IVF birth, the IVF field has expanded to include a growing range of artificial reproduction methods.

By the early 1980s IVF was being touted as another great service to humankind, as another great step in human control of reproduction, meaning scientist-controlled reproduction. Among the benefits of IVF and human embryo research, IVF advocates list: (i) improving the treatment of infertility in both females and males; (ii) offering a socially better option to adoption; (iii) gaining knowledge about congenital (at birth) conditions; (iv) reducing genetic abnormality in offspring; and (v) developing more effective forms of contraception. After this first round of promised benefits, we learn that scientists also 'need' embryos for reasons which have nothing whatsoever to do with reproduction. Medical researchers wish to use human embryos to grow tissue for transplants and treating conditions such as Parkinson's Disease and diabetes, to test drugs, and to study how cells work, especially the genetic mechanisms that occur in embryonic cells. The medical/scientific scope seems limitless.

The most enthusiastic advocates articulate the ultimate meaning of all this. US biologist and policy commentator Clifford Grobstein states outright that external human fertilisation (IVF by another name) 'raises the possibility that some day we shall be able to influence the biological nature of our own species' and 'the present period may be viewed . . . as the beginning of a second great human transition' (Grobstein, 1981, p. xi). Grobstein's dream of a scientist-directed evolution and transformation in human relations is not a new idea; prominent scientists such as embryologist Conrad H. Waddington of Edinburgh University and geneticist Hermann J. Muller of Indiana University had articulated the dream in *The Humanist Frame*, published in 1961, seventeen years before the first 'test-tube' baby was born and twenty years before Grobstein's book, *From Chance to Purpose: An Appraisal of External Human Fertilisation* (see Chapter 7). Though Grobstein prefers the accuracy of the term *external human fertilisation*, rather than *in vitro* fertilisation, he has missed a point. It is actually external-*to-woman* fertilisation. The scientific dream of a scientist-directed evolution must happen on women's bodies, where eggs and embryos come from.

This book, then, is primarily about the accountability of scientists, especially medical scientists, to women. It is about the motivations of scientists pursuing knowledge about women's reproduction. It is about the values underlying reproductive science and technology. It is about the further shift in emphasis in obstetrics and gynaecology to a scientific approach to women's reproduction. It is about the effect on women of the new reproductive and genetic technologies being used on us in the name of medical therapy.

The accountability of scientists and doctors is crucial to understanding what is happening in the reproductive technology area. Scientific concepts about women's reproduction, and the new reproductive technologies, have transformed both the practice of medicine and our everyday consciousness of fertility, pregnancy and heredity (most obviously, the relationship between genes and traits). Further, professional 'experts' – philosophers, ethicists, doctors, social scientists, lawyers, judges, government inquiries – have for the most part accepted a scientific assessment of what is meant by reproduction. Scientific concepts and technologies are being used as the basis for setting the standards of making moral and social judgements about human reproductive practice, and so about women's reproductive behaviour. In the past, this was the role of religion. Today science acts as a kind of religious belief in industrialised societies, where scientific knowledge is considered superior, 'objective', and closer to the truth.

Terminology

The following are brief descriptions of the general terms used throughout this book: *in vitro* fertilisation (IVF), IVF practitioners, technology, the new reproductive technologies, genetic engineering and reproductive engineering. The meanings of more particular terms, such as cloning and embryo transfer, will be given in subsequent chapters as they arise. The glossary also describes these terms, and so may be used for quick reference.

In vitro fertilisation is a scientific term. *In vitro*, literally 'in glass', describes biological processes which are made to occur outside the living body, and in laboratory apparatus. By contrast the term *in vivo* describes biological processes which are observed occurring in their natural environment within the living organism. In IVF, the egg and sperm are placed in a laboratory dish in a culture medium which contains nutrients and substances necessary for growth. The prerequisite for IVF is removing eggs from women's bodies, usually by the administration of powerful fertility drugs and hormones to stimulate our ovaries and control our menstrual cycles; fertility monitoring with ultrasound; removal of ripe eggs from our ovaries[2]; embryo transfer from laboratory dish to our wombs; and if pregnancy results possibly more hormones, ultrasound scanning, amniocentesis and usually Caesarean section birth. The risks of the IVF procedures to women and offspring have never been fully investigated before being used on women as a treatment for fertility problems.

Throughout this book I use the words *IVF methods* to mean all the methods associated with removing women's eggs and using them, whether or not the removed egg is fertilised, and whether or not eggs and embryos *in vitro* are destined for clinical use on women or for research. This is not always the best way to refer to the range of *in vitro* procedures. For example, an embryo conceived *in vivo* (in a women's body) can be flushed out of her womb, at which point it becomes an *in vitro* embryo. However, the ability to remove women's eggs, and then grow and fertilise them in the laboratory is central to the new 'artificial reproduction' technologies. IVF has made feasible the use of human embryos for research, since now researchers have access to eggs from women in IVF programmes. Also the use of IVF in women encourages other interventions including surrogacy, genetic engineering of embryos, the further development of artificial wombs, and human embryo research projects. The use of IVF on women opened the door to using all these other, related reproductive and genetic technologies.

I tend to use scientific phrases (e.g. *in vivo* and human reproduction) when reporting the work or paraphrasing the words of medical scientists, even as I try to decode their language. I want to reflect accurately the message coming from IVF doctors and scientists, yet not let their language set the agenda. This has proved awkward. The scientific language itself is insidious.

IVF practitioners come in many guises. There are the reproductive physiologists like Robert Edwards who take part in clinical IVF on women as well as 'pure' research on animals and women's eggs. There are medical doctors like gynaecologist Patrick Steptoe who carry out clinical applications of IVF on women and who collaborate with IVF researchers. There are researchers (embryologists, geneticists, physiologists, immunologists, endocrinologists, and so on) who carry out research on eggs and embryos and genes *in vitro* (that is, outside the living organisms). Some of them experiment solely on animals, some work on women's body parts, some work on both. Many experiment with embryos and fetuses which do not originate from *in vitro* fertilisation: some work with human fetuses obtained from abortions. I consider all these doctors and scientists *medical scientists*. Even those IVF doctors who presumably do not carry out research are still taking part in scientific experiments and endeavours based in high technology, and so acting as medical scientists. Likewise, those research scientists who experiment on embryos or older fetuses are involved in medical research, even when they do not carry out medical application on women. This is not my personal assessment, but the view of governments and funding bodies. Much public and private 'medical research' money is granted to biologists, biochemists, physicists, and others for so-called 'pure' research which has little obvious clinical (medical) application.

Technology in its simplest definition is the practical application of scientific knowledge. This is not an adequate definition, however. A technology is not merely a technique or a machine. A technology is not a thing. It is a system that includes organisational factors, aims and values, as well as 'technical' techniques. In considering technology we must consider where the 'technical' techniques come from, why they are considered valuable, and how they are administered. Technology is political.

The interrelationship between (natural) science and technology is fundamental. By technology I mean *science-based technology* and technology-based science. The science–technology relationship is particular to each technology, and it depends on an entwining of factors, such as ideology[3], economic interests, military interests, and so on. This is an important point. IVF could not have been developed in a vacuum by, say, some individual working in a garage with a few simple tools. As research scientists, Robert Edwards and colleagues work within a highly organised and developed scientific community, which functions within specific social and cultural conditions. To proceed with their sophisticated research in keeping eggs, embryos and fetuses alive outside living female bodies, these researchers must have access to laboratories, equipment, supplies, and experimental animals; those researching 'human IVF' must have access to women. The research scientists pursuing these experiments perceive the scientific worth of IVF and related procedures in the context of the science that went before them and the science that is going on around them (Chapters 5 and 6). Finally, they must direct so-called practical application of their work in some way that is acceptable to the state and presumably to the public.

The term *new reproductive technologies* (NRTs) is recent. The NRTs include IVF, embryo transfer, sex preselection, genetic engineering of embryos, cloning (making genetically identical individuals) and more. They are new because they are relatively recent developments, based on new capabilities. But they come from the same scientific approach to reproduction control which brought us 'old' reproductive technologies such as hormonal contraceptives (the Pill) in the 1950s and 60s, and pre-natal screening (amniocentesis) by the late 1960s.

Reproductive technologies, old and new, include genetic technologies. Genetics is the science aimed at finding out what genes are and how they work (see Chapter 6). Genes were once defined as 'units of heredity', since the genes in the egg and sperm cells carry genetic information from one generation to the next. The information genes carry is necessary for embryo development and functioning of the living body. In the 1940s and 50s, the first modern genetic technologies emerged. These were techniques for looking at chromosomes (where genes are packaged in the cell) with microscopes, and biochemical methods for measuring the presence of gene products (proteins) in blood or amniotic fluid.

The connection between genetic technology and reproductive technology is important. Not all genetic technology today is directly related to reproduction, and not all reproductive technologies are directly concerned with genetics. But the new reproductive and genetic technologies exist in a symbiotic relationship. When I talk about the new reproductive technologies overall, I include the related genetic technologies.

Renate Klein describes *reproductive technology* as the full range of biomedical/technical interferences during the process of procreation, whether aimed at producing a child or preventing/terminating pregnancy (Klein, 1985). Reproductive technology then includes the new reproductive technologies such as IVF or cloning (a genetic technology), but also modern contraceptives, sterilisation techniques, genetic screening (a genetic technology), and so on.

Genetic engineering, the most daunting expression of all, refers to a variety of methods available to scientists for altering the genetic make-up of living things. Genetic engineering may be aimed at the level of cells, or directly at the level of genes within the cell. The term was coined in the 1960s when new techniques allowed scientists to produce genetic changes in organisms by manipulating cells, where the genetic material (DNA, what genes are made of) is located. By the early 1970s proteins called 'restriction enzymes' were discovered, allowing scientists to alter genes directly. The 'restriction enzymes' allowed a kind of 'cut and paste' transection for removing pieces of genetic material from one organism, and then inserting the pieces into the genetic material of another. It is considered the most important genetic engineering method for use in industry and medicine. I use the term genetic engineering in a broad sense to mean any of these scientific methods aimed at manipulating the genetic make-up of living things. (By contrast, some textbooks and articles limit the use of the phrase 'genetic engineering' to mean manipulation of genes on the molecular level with restriction enzymes.)

Another often used term is *eugenics*, the science of improving the human 'stock', championed by the English scientist Sir Francis Galton (1822–1911). By eugenics I mean any method of selective breeding used for population control, whether for quantity control or quality control.

Prospects in *reproductive engineering* follow from the new reproductive and genetic technologies. Because medical scientists can manipulate women's fertility by manipulating eggs and embryos both in a woman's womb and in laboratories, and because changing genetic make-up is now possible, they can alter the 'products' of reproduction. Scientists and governments recognised the reproductive engineering aspects of IVF methods early on. In 1972, reproductive technology was ominously defined in the *Journal of the American Medical Association* and repeated in a US government publication as,

> covering anything to do with the manipulation of gametes [eggs or sperm] or the fetus, for whatever purpose, from conception other than by sexual union, to treatment of disease *in utero*, to the ultimate manufacture of a human being to exact specifications . . . Thus the earliest procedure . . . is artificial insemination; next . . . artificial fertilisation . . . next artificial implantation . . . in the future extracorporeal gestation [artificial womb] . . . and finally, what is popularly meant by (reproductive) engineering, the production – or better, the biological manufacture – of a human being to desired specification.[4]

The definition is indicative of the dominant discussions and debates on reproductive and genetic technology in that there are *no women mentioned as the subject of human reproduction*. There are eggs and sperm, embryos and fetuses, wombs and scientific techniques, there are body parts and biological processes but there are no women as whole human beings. This lack of recognising women's active presence in reproduction recurs in medical textbooks, in scientific articles, and in government reports on the issues. They inevitably speak in terms of body parts, such as 'man's eggs' or 'human placenta' or 'human reproduction' when expressly describing distinctly female physiology and biochemistry. As we will see, this kind of language and attitude masks the fact that women are the central subjects of 'human reproduction' and the central subjects on whom the new reproductive technologies are used. It allows medical scientists with the backing of the state to proceed with reproductive engineering projects without accountability to women.

Loss of women's identity in the scientific model

Reproduction is not simply a biological process. Women do not breed like cows, Maria Mies writes. 'Women's activity in producing children and milk is understood as truly human, i.e. a conscious, social activity' (Mies, 1981, p. 12).

Mies underlines that women have in the past experienced and observed their reproduction, and passed on the knowledge they have gained to their daughters. Women's experiences of the productivity of our whole bodies affects who we are, and how we relate to the world. This is not a biologistic argument, that is one that reduces women's behaviour to biology. It is a rejection of the false split between the 'purely' biological and the social. It is an affirmation of women's sensuous reproduction and our bodily human existence in the world. And it is a rejection of the notion that women are passive incubators during pregnancy and birth. Women have and do acquire a vast knowledge of fertility and reproduction from experience.

This knowledge, women's experiential knowledge of reproduction, is considered 'unscientific' and not credible. For example, a London midwife pointed out that pregnant women who can pinpoint the exact date of intercourse as the time they became pregnant are met with disbelief by medical doctors, even when pregnancy testing technology (ultrasound scanning) is giving them obviously incorrect information.[5]

Scientists learn to work in a 'disinterested' relationship to nature, where an observer (the scientist) is supposedly removed and outside the object of study (nature). In the area of 'human reproduction', that object of study is woman (see Chapter 5). In the words of the prestigious international science journal *Nature* (1983, p. 735), the aim of IVF/human embryo research is 'to improve, so to speak, on nature'. More accurately, to improve, so to speak, on women.

Leading US IVF practitioner Howard Jones (1985) voiced a similar message: 'Medically, human reproduction is surprisingly inefficient.' What he was actually talking about was the statistical chances of a fertile woman becoming pregnant. As an expert witness for a US Congressional hearing on Human Embryo Transfer in August 1984, Jones used the inefficiency 'problem' to argue the case for allowing IVF/human embryo research.

US gynaecologist and research scientist Luigi Mastroianni warned against the premature use of IVF on women in the 1970s. But in the philosophical–scientific commentary applauding artificial reproduction technologies entitled *From Chance to Purpose*

18   *Beyond Conception*

(1981), Clifford Grobstein noted that Mastroianni's concern centred on the risks to the fetus, not with 'the potential mother, who, of course, is the actual subject of the procedure' (p. 26). Grobstein concluded, 'this reflects the general medical consensus that *the risk to the patient is minimal* . . . The consensus takes into account, also, the obviously strong motivation of sterile couples to overcome almost any obstacle to have a child of their own – *including considerable risk*' (pp. 26–7, my emphasis). How can IVF be both risky and not risky? Mastroianni now heads the IVF programme at the University of Pennsylvania Hospital in Philadelphia, although the primate studies he called for were never done.

Having dismissed the risks to women in the early pages of this book, without any substantial medical evidence that the procedures were safe, Grobstein then pondered in lengthy detail the human subjectivity of embryos and the scientific wonders of *in vitro* fertilisation and genetic engineering. His identification of the 'potential mother' (a woman) as the 'actual subject' was mere lip service. His naming of the woman undergoing IVF as the 'potential mother' was not even accurate since the success rate is extremely low and few women leave an IVF programme with live babies (see Chapters 3 and 4).

Science makes medicine more prestigious and more 'exact'. The Western medical model is often criticised for seeing diseases and parts of bodies instead of seeing the patient as a whole person. But in the area of 'human reproduction' women's loss of identity is even more profound. Pregnancy and childbirth are not illness, yet medical technologies such as ultrasound, and now the new reproductive technologies are being used on more and more healthy women, carrying women's fertility further into the domain of medical expertise.

Furthermore, taking the high-tech scientific route to women's and men's fertility problems has pre-empted a substantive discussion of why some women and men who cannot reproduce experience a life crisis, what motherhood and non-motherhood means, why fertility problems are increasing among women and men globally, and how fertility problems can be prevented. By the logic of technology (a Maria Mies phrase), IVF is promoted as a cure for infertility and a means to avoid genetic defect, but the medical and social causes of fertility problems and congenital conditions are being ignored (see Chapters 4 and 8).

What is most often not understood is that the emphasis on reproductive technology is about a particular kind of control of human reproductive capacities. The technology-minded circumvent iatrogenic (doctor-induced) causes of women's fertility problems such as the IUD and excessive abdominal surgery on a case-by-case basis by looking to IVF as a 'cure'; and instead of recognising poor health care, nutrition, and other environmental factors as a major cause of congenital conditions, for which there is medical evidence, they are emphasising the genetic manipulation of embryos approach. In the context of gross mismanagement of primary health care and lack of recognition of environmental factors which lead to reproductive problems in women and men, the overall lack of concern for women's health becomes even more obvious.

Let me stress that the use of the new reproductive technologies is expanding to include more and more women, not just a few women. As Professor Jerome Strauss, Director of the Division of Reproductive Biology at the Hospital of the University of Pennsylvania, explained, *IVF changed the course of obstetrics and gynaecology.*[6] IVF's impact is in the whole area of women's reproductive capacities; it is not just an infertility management procedure. Among others, Professor Mark Ferguson of Manchester University suggested why, in future, IVF might be used as a preferred mode of reproduction by couples who do not have fertility problems. He explained that embryos could be frozen for spare parts, for example their cells could generate new teeth. He offered, 'Individuals may choose to reproduce by IVF so as to have a bank af spare parts for their offspring when the latter begin to suffer from diseases or injuries' (*The Guardian*, 1987d). And IVF is crucial for academic careers. Dr Gary D. Hodgen, who resigned his post as chief of pregnancy research at the National Institutes of Health because the US government will not fund 'human embryo' research, said to a US Congressional hearing, 'No mentor of young physicians and scientists beginning their academic careers in reproductive medicine can deny the central importance of *in vitro* fertilisation-embryo transfer research' (*Current Contents*, 1984).

Balancing act: the status of embryos and the status of science

When the possibility of using IVF on women became apparent in the early 1970s, medical, legal, and moral questions were raised within the context of ethics debates. Ethicists, scientists, doctors, theologians, lawyers, policy-makers, social scientists, psychologists, and politicians have had a say on ethical committees set up by hospitals, private foundations and governments. There are old moral concerns, like the 'status of the embryo', and there are new concerns, like 'egg donation'.

In the 'expert' ethical debate over IVF, the dominant moral concerns are the status of the embryo, interference in marriage, and a fear that scientists doing IVF might disrupt the ties that bind society, such as the meaning of paternity and motherhood. The balancing term, the term which qualifies old norms about embryos and privacy in marriage, is a purported need for scientific 'progress'. In a paper presented to the Eugenics Society in London, in 1982, Robert Edwards wrote, 'I believe that the need for knowledge is greater than the respect to be accorded to an early embryo' (Edwards, 1983a, p. 104). Professor Roger Short, another British research scientist, championed the use of IVF on women in 1978. He thought that preliminary primate studies would be too time consuming, saying 'it would seem wrong to hold up progress until the information was available'.[7]

The two dominating preoccupations in the mainstream professional debate on IVF issues are embryos and scientific knowledge ('progress'). The naming of issues and their meaning by scientists and professional ethicists set the agenda for their ethics debates. As the magazine *New Scientist* declared in 1982 (a, p. 290): 'The important ethical question is: should scientists conduct research on live human embryos? When do embryos become people?' The tension in the professional 'expert' debate over the NRTs is not about *how* science is being conducted nor about the use of women's bodies for experimental material. The tensions are between ideology and technology. That is, how far should scientists be allowed to go in altering traditional social relations in the area of reproduction and kinship? And how much authority over women's reproduction should IVF practitioners themselves enjoy?

The two big issues, status of embryos and need for scientific inquiry, are not inevitable. They come from a certain way of perceiving women and our reproductive capacities. For example, the journal *Nature* equates removing a wife's eggs with procuring a husband's sperm. They argued, 'uneasiness that the ova [eggs] are obtained artificially by a relatively simple procedure is understandable but indefensibly irrational, given the widespread and apparently acceptable practice of artifical insemination with a husband's sperm' (*Nature*, 1982, p. 475). They ignore the obviously different processes involved in procuring eggs and sperm. The hormone and drug regimens, the surgery, the removal of women's internal body parts, the months and even years of a woman's physical and emotional commitment to IVF treatment which affects everything else she is doing means nothing to them; to suggest that it means something is 'indefensibly irrational'.

This is what I mean by women not being a presence in scientific reproduction. Invasive, technological intervention is the only means to gain access to women's eggs and that means tampering with our biochemistry and physiology and the whole living system of our bodies (see Chapter 3). Men's sperm is not equivalent. There is no violent disruption of life processes to acquire sperm, as is necessary to acquire eggs. By the logic *Nature* used, women's role at this stage of reproduction is reduced to that of men's. Women mean nothing in this sort of logic.

Embryos mean something, but paradoxically. On the one hand, IVF practitioners assure everyone that they have due respect for embryos. On the other hand, these same IVF practitioners must handle and inevitably destroy or discard human embryos. The lack of discussion by scientists about this paradox is an insult to women. In Britain, for example, since the criminalisation of abortion in 1803 the law in practice maintains that the interests of embryos supersede women's self-determination over our own bodies. The liberalisation of the abortion law by the Abortion Act 1967 does not remove elements of criminality and medical–legal control of women's reproductive behaviour. Doctors and the state will have the authority to 'protect' embryos from women. A woman who wishes to have a legal abortion in Britain must receive the permission of two doctors, and her reasons must fit into the criteria set out in the Abortion Act. We depend on both the decisions (and prejudices) of individual doctors and on the availablity of doctors who are willing to offer abortion services. For example, the same doctor who might encourage an abortion if the fetus is shown by pre-natal screening to be afflicted with some condition, may refuse to give permission for other reasons.

Meanwhile, various medical and scientific bodies and the British Government's Warnock Inquiry into IVF issues are willing to allow human embryo research at least up to fourteen days after fertilisation in the laboratory dish. Why do embryo interests supersede women's interests, but the interests of medical science supersede embryo interests?, Why are scientists allowed to argue for their authority to handle and manipulate embryos because of some greater 'good', which they define, while a pregnant woman who might wish to have an abortion is denied self-determination over her own body and life? Why do scientists ignore this moral paradox, as if it is reasonable and just? Doctors and research scientists must understand this point, but choose to ignore it as irrelevant to their discussion of the ethics of IVF.[8] It is another indication of the invisibility of women.

IVF advocates are willing to keep the ethical discussion revolving around embryos. Ignoring women and talking in terms of embryos is morally less problematic than admitting that women are the subjects of 'human IVF' and 'human embryo' experimentation. It is much easier to deal with the ethics of experimentation with embryos rather than the ethics of experimenting with women's bodies. The message of those individuals and groups who advocate the new reproductive technologies is that scientific knowledge about embryos (rather than pregnancy: what goes on in women's bodies) is essential to help infertile couples, to prevent congenital 'defect', to create 'ideal' contraceptives, and so on. To carry out their 'essential' work, medical scientists must have access to women's body parts.

Ignoring women as the subject of pregnancy, the 'experts' are left with embryos. Proponents of IVF, most especially the IVF practitioners themselves, cannot dismiss the embryo as totally without special status even as they recommend experimenting on and discarding embryos. If they did not voice great moral concern for (some) embryos, they would appear as immoral Dr Frankensteins and lose their status and authority. If they were true to their scientific convictions that embryos and fetuses should be available to researchers and that a fertilised egg (an embryo) is no more special than, say, unfertilised eggs, then they would be left with having to admit that in fact it is women who are the subject of their experimentation. So, they play politics with the meaning of the embryo. This has taken many forms:

— IVF, which involves the manipulation and inevitable destruction of embryos, must be reconciled to the traditional ethic of the embryo. Research on embryos helps future embryos, the logic goes. Most IVF practitioners concede that the embryo has some level of special status, but they make a distinction between those embryos which are worthy of special consideration, and those embryos which should have no special status, and thus be experimented on.

— Among those they play politics with are anti-abortionists. One argument put forward by IVF practitioners Carl Wood in Australia, Jack Glatt in England, and Dominico Garcia in Italy is that IVF is not the destruction of life, as in abortion, but the creation of life (see pp. 38, 81).

— In Britain, the Voluntary Licensing Authority, a medical/science sponsored body which oversees IVF practice and research, renamed the early embryo a 'pre-embryo' to coincide exactly with the time limit placed on 'human embryo' research.

In the end, advocates of the new reproductive technologies are balancing what have become the two major subjects in the 'public' discussion on IVF and human embryo research: the status of the embryo and the status of science. They would argue that women's interests are taken into account by scientific 'progressive' interests. This is the same kind of thinking that assumes that women's interests are served by the wonders of science, without any consideration of the harm that so-called advances such as powerful hormonal contraceptives, or the miscarriage drug DES, has had on women (see Chapter 4). This kind of thinking subsumes women's interests to the interests of medical science, population engineers, pharmaceutical companies that profit from the proliferation of new technologies, and of course the new biotechnology industry.

Anti-abortionists do not qualify the sanctity of the embryo in the way such advocates of human embryo research do. They oppose human embryo research absolutely, not because it harms women, but because they view the embryo as the person who is being harmed by these technologies. The anti-abortionists accept a separation between women and embryo in a particular way, different from the way IVF advocates separate women and embryos (or fetuses). As feminist philosopher Janice Raymond (1987) drives home, in *Fetalists and Feminists: They Are Not the Same*, the position of anti-abortionists subsumes the interests and rights of women to the 'interests' and 'rights' of the developing fetus.

Both sorts of fetal-centred thinking, whether coming from advocates of IVF and the other new reproductive technologies or from anti-abortionists, function to keep women's human identity subsumed and subservient to someone else's interests. The anti-abortion lobbies in various countries are notorious for their desire to maintain the ideology of the nuclear family, with women's social role and legal rights narrowly defined within that ideology. Progressive IVF advocates, though they appear to be at odds with traditional mores, are in fact creating their own brand of fetalism, which considers embryos as so necessary to scientific progress that women should be willing to place our bodies in their hands.

Also, as we will see in subsequent chapters, the practice of IVF on women is being carried out, not with respect to women's health care needs, but as a means to assert those very institutions which anti-abortionists have been trying to salvage. IVF is being offered as a medical therapy but only for couples living together, not for women. Eligibility for IVF in most countries is restricted to married women or women living with men in 'stable' relationships, in '*de facto* marriages' as they say. IVF practitioners are willing to play politics with the meaning of infertility to fit into a framework which serves patriarchal social conditions. When a women is married (or living with a man in a marital relationship), her infertility or her partner's infertility is considered a medical condition. All other women who have fertility problems, lesbians and single women, are not eligible for such medical 'treatment'. Obviously, IVF is not only being used as a medical treatment but as a social treatment.[9]

By contrast, no authorities are willing to offer women by ourselves (all women) the most basic means of securing healthy, autonomous conditions to procreate, such as economic and social security, adequate primary health care, and protection of women's rights as free social beings.

Whatever gains towards sexual and reproductive freedom women have made since the 1960s, the emphasis on reproductive engineering is marginalising those gains. Certainly, in Britain the legal rights of unmarried mothers established in the 1970s appear precarious if the state is going to endorse the social *superiority* of the wife/husband couple, as it has in the Warnock Report, the report of the official government sponsored investigation on IVF issues (see Chapter 8). This has implications for all women, and on practical levels. Governments are regulating the use of IVF as a reproductive technique, and any social and moral presumptions they endorse with respect to women's sexuality, motherhood, and embryos will become criteria for judging all women's reproductive behaviour.

IVF advocates often cite another argument to promote the use of IVF on women, the 'right' to procreate. Robert Edwards (1974) set up this argument for future IVF practitioners when he reminded readers of the *Quarterly Review of Biology* that the 'right to have children is stated in various international declarations on human rights' (p. 10). This 'right' is repeatedly stated in ethics reports and in scientific papers on IVF. From there follows a 'right to treatment'. Edwards took it further, noting 'the rights and *duty* of scientists and doctors to study embryos' (Edwards, 1983a, p. 102, my emphasis). That statement is not far from inferring that IVF/human embryo research is an ethical imperative! More accurately, experimentation using women's bodies is an ethical imperative.

Technology-knowledge

Western industrialised countries are called technological societies, 'knowledge-based' societies, where true knowledge is considered scientific knowledge, and where science entails technology as the 'tools' of knowledge acquisition. This very specific kind of knowledge, grounded in a particular way of viewing the world and utilising nature, is being used as the basis for making ethical judgements about the new reproductive technologies, as if it is 'neutral' knowledge of biological events, bringing untold benefits in its wake.

IVF advocates have accommodated the 'status of the embryo' by defining it in terms of scientific knowledge (what scientists know about embryos). They have appropriated ethics as dependent on scientific knowledge (what scientists know).

According to Robert Edwards (1983a), ethics are based on a rational set of values, capable of scientific verification or impartial judgement whenever possible. (Rationality is the hallmark of a scientific approach.) As science advances, he explained in his presentation to the Eugenics Society in 1982, standards of judgement and behaviour established at one period may have to change with new discoveries and thinking. Clifford Grobstein urges similarly. Scientific rationality thus becomes the guiding principle for ethical standards. To these scientists, forgers of a new and 'better' morality, it is then the duty of the rest of us to keep up with science. If you do not agree, you are irrational, uninformed, unknowledgeable, uncooperative, and prejudiced. Edwards was quoted in the popular magazine *New Scientist*, 'What do ethics mean . . . a standard of behaviour and activity that you decide upon for various reasons. Some are codified in law but in our field there is no law . . . Scientists make ethics as they go along' (Yanchinski, 1982).

Advocates of the new reproductive technologies in other professions – ethicists, theologians, policy-makers, population planners and social scientists - recognise this as a legitimate approach. Mary Warnock, a philosopher and the chair of the British Government's Committee of Inquiry which investigated IVF issues, concurs that today's scientific knowledge about embryos should inform society's moral judgements about human embryo research. She is in favour of embryo research, and she is also preoccupied with the 'status of the embryo', not recognising women as the central subject of embryology (what happens in pregnancy). At a lecture delivered in 1987 at the University of York on the philosophical topic 'Toleration', she suggested that scientific information about embryos brings the moral question into line. She noted that some of us know that the early embryo is but a few cells, undifferentiated, not yet an 'individual' in the biological sense. At one stage in the talk she acknowledged that the question of the personhood of embryos was a moral question, a matter of value judgement. But at two other junctures she looked to the *scientific facts*, as if they are neutral facts, for direction in making that value judgement.

So, biological 'facts' are a basis of ethics. Biological knowledge about embryos, brought to us by scientific experimentation on embryos, sets the ethics of IVF and human embryo experimentation. It sounds tautological because it is.

Similarly, scientific concepts of genetics and 'genetic identity' are swiftly becoming the most important defining aspect of human relations and control of reproduction (see Chapters 6, 7, 8). Joseph Fletcher, an ethicist, theologian and great believer in the superiority of artificial reproduction, published his affirmation of reproductive engineering in *The Ethics of Genetic Control: Ending Reproductive Roulette* (1974). Fletcher favours the limitation of the right to procreate to genetically 'fit' women, once stating, 'There are more Typhoid Marys carrying genetic disease than infectious disease' (quoted in Milunsky and Annas, 1980, pp. x–xi).

IVF scientists seem to have it both ways: scientific knowledge is neutral (never bad), and science is positively good (never bad). By the science-is-neutral argument, science and technology remains 'technical' and value-free. Robert Edwards was quoted in the press as saying, 'Science is being attacked unfairly, because science is neutral' (Prentice, 1984). By this rationale IVF does not in itself harm women; rather using it in the 'wrong' way harms women. It is a baldly naïve argument, masking the physical risks to women of IVF, and its emotional and social costs.

Reflecting the science-is-good ('progress') belief, the journal *Nature* (1985b) argued that the British Government should allow IVF and human embryo research whose benefits would only become apparent with time. IVF apologists in Britain continually repeated this statement in public. Their message is, trust that reproductive technologies will benefit society and individuals *eventually*. Yet we already know that infertility could be managed *now* by better primary health care for women, screening for pelvic inflammatory disease and cervical cancer, by securing a higher standard of hygiene and nutrition for poor women, by cleaning up the workplace from environmental hazards that cause infertility in women and men, and congenital health problems in infants. These aspects do not fit into the pursuit and application of technology-knowledge, however.

Finally, there is the point of view of scientists who find ethics a bother, such as Dr Michael Birnbaum, founder of Surrogate Mothering Ltd in Philadelphia (USA). He later became director of a new IVF clinic after his surrogacy business collapsed. Birnbaum was quoted in a Philadelphia newspaper: 'The ethical questions are always there, but the minute we stop doing something because of ethics, we stop going forward and start going backward' (Mezzacappa, 1986).

Such is the power of the scientific world view which sees 'progress' as a continuous motion forward. I think the difference between Birnbaum's attitude and Mary Warnock's attitude is revealing. Warnock would mould the ethics to scientific knowledge, while Birnbaum is not fussed about the ethics. Neither view recognises respect for women's integrity as a basis for making ethical judgements about invasive procedures on women's bodies.

Liability and informed consent

The existence of embryos outside a woman's body raises question of legal ownership, legal authority, and responsibility towards embryos. Typically, it has not raised the question about responsibility and accountability to woman, from whom eggs and embryos and other internal body parts are extracted, and on whom the entire IVF procedure is carried out. Since the 1970s Robert Edwards has co-authored several articles with lawyers calling for a legal framework under which IVF practitioners could practise. His stated concern is protecting the researcher from liability in the legal sense. In a 1975 paper on various kinds of medical science intervention into reproduction, Edwards and co-author Ian Kennedy warned (threatened?) that treatment could be withheld if doctors became alarmed over the lack of adequate guidelines as to their legal position and responsibility (Kennedy and Edwards, 1975).

Edwards recognised early on the need for parental consent. In a 1984 article, he and barrister Margaret Puxon concluded that IVF practitioners must receive parental consent to create and handle embryos, and that in carrying out their work 'the best interests of the child' is the paramount concern (Edwards and Puxon, 1984). Now, this stress on the interests of the child is predictable. The 'best interests of the child' is the standard that prevails in current family law. Legal and moral judgements, in courts and other social institutions, always consider that the star criterion. However, it is not as straightforward as it reads, since of course the 'best interests of the child' is not so easily determined and is in most cases a value judgement.

The legal concern over the 'best interests of the child' prompts issues of illegitimacy, inheritance, paternity, maternal fitness, and that includes social judgements as to women's sexuality or economic status, and now even the status of maternity itself in cases of 'surrogacy' and 'egg donation' (see Chapter 8). Even when the 'best interests of the child' works in favour of a woman, as in some examples of custody cases, the term is precarious for women. It depends on definitions of motherhood (the 'natural' mother–child bond, marital stability, etc) which tend to define certain kinds of women as 'fit' mothers, and other kinds of women (lesbians, single women, poor women, even feminist women) as 'unfit' mothers (Hanmer, 1985). The various permutations of IVF, like 'egg donation' and 'embryo donation', are similarly being measured in terms of how it effects traditional family relations with actually little concern for what the long-term effects will be on the resulting children. It is clear that the 'best interests of children' concept is not simply about the best interests of children.

IVF advocates have coopted the legal concept 'the best interests of the child' to argue in favour of experimentation on embryos. The journal *Nature* (1985c) argued awkwardly that human embryo research aimed at studying congenital abnormality is in 'the best interests of children in general'. They stretched the point further to argue, 'And is there not, in any case, a proper sense in which the interests of children in general may supervene over the interests of individual embryos?' (*Nature*, 1985b). I suspect they could take that rationale further to argue that women must give up our eggs and bodies to science in the best interests of children who will benefit from the knowledge gained.

Everyone on biomedical ethics committees insits on 'informed consent' from patients, or in the case of IVF, the prospective parents (that is the couple, not the women undergoing the medical procedures). But informed consent works to protect IVF practitioners and hospitals, not the identified parents of the embryo, certainly not women who are the real subjects of IVF intervention.[10] The official informed consent agreement recommended to IVF clinics in Britain by the Voluntary Licensing Authority (VLA) is a case in point. The couple signing the form agree to, among other things, 'preparation of the woman by the administration of hormones and other drugs . . . maintenance of pre-embryos [sic] resulting from such fertilisation . . . *selection by the medical staff* of the most suitable pre-embryos for such replacment (MRC/RCOG VLA, 1986, pp. 41–2, my emphasis).

Astute scientists have realised that 'informed consent' protects them. British physiologist Professor Robert A. McCance (1977) called the setting up of ethical committees to control biomedical practices on humans an unfortunate consequence of bad publicity in the 1960s. McCance carried out research on 'immature' human fetuses at Cambridge in the 1960s. He has been a vocal proponent of the investigator's right to exercise his or her own conscience on matters of experimenting with human fetuses, premature babies, children and adults. He lamented over the ties that bind the researcher.

> Meantime, progress is bound to slow down, unless of course, as has happened so often in this country, mutually satisfactory catch phrases, conventions and compromises such as 'informed consent' free the human physiologists from the shackles of a politically minded and usually uncooperative public. (McCance, 1977, p. 155)

As all medical ethicists know, the hierarchical doctor–patient or scientist–subject relationship counters an easy acceptance of informed consent. Medical scientists have access in operating rooms to women's body parts. Women seeking medical help, like all people tagged 'patients', will act in ways that work towards our receiving the treatment we seek. Women on IVF programmes say this, as Christine Crowe (1987a) reported from discussions with women in Australian IVF programmes; and professional ethicists have admitted this too. On the rare occasion, a medical scientist does. As an 'expert' witness to the US Ethics Advisory Board in 1978, Luigi Mastroianni warned that infertility patients (women) might be influenced to take part in risky research by their desire to have children. Medical ethicists also pointed out in the early debates that many patients (women) would be reluctant to disappoint doctors.

Yet the argument prevails, if we do not want to participate in an experiment, we do not have to. But although there may be many women who freely and gladly wish to give up eggs and embryos to science, there is the question of why invasive surgery and removal of women's internal body parts is necessary for 'progress'. Also, and most obviously, there is the predicament of women who want to be accepted onto IVF programmes, and women undergoing gynaecological surgery who feel the need to keep the surgeons happy. These women are left with little choice. On top of that is the power in Western societies of the scientist's word. The message we are hearing from the medical and science establishments is that doctors and researchers *must* have access to women's body parts or else they will not be able to help women have healthy babies. Again, the logic of technology.

A feminist ethic

IVF advocates *versus* the anti-technology anti-abortionists appear as the congealed 'sides' of the ethics debate, *as if* they were the *total* debate. There has been little recognition publicly of a woman-centred analysis which criticises reproductive and genetic technologies. This is changing.

In West Germany and Australia, a concerted feminist critical response to the NRTs has appeared in the media since the early 1980s, effecting a certain amount of recognition from politicians and governments. However, feminist activists are wary that the stricter controls and regulation implemented in these two countries are acting more as a public tranquilliser than a safeguard to women's rights and integrity. Much government control to date has been a means to regularise experimentation in this area, and make it formally acceptable to the public. For example, the ban on embryo research in West Germany is qualified by their allowing 'essential' medical research. But as I pointed out in the Introduction, much 'basic' or 'pure' research on biological systems passes as medical research today.

In questioning the worth of reproductive and genetic technology feminists are not playing the role of anti-technology terrorists. We are not even playing on the stage of the supposedly 'public' debate that does not even acknowledge women as women, as whole human autonomous beings.

Feminist resistance to the new reproductive technologies can be understood in the context of the women's health movement, where the conditions are being created for *women-centred* health care and medical research. Not embryo-centred, not 'progress'-centred, but women-centred.

A feminist ethic holds that the aims of reproductive health care and medical research must be focused on what will serve women best, not what will serve scientists best. For instance, feminist health centres and clinics around the world are organised around the principle that women are the primary subject of our own fertility, pregnancy and childbirth. The resurgence of midwifery and home birth in Western countries is another example, where pregnancy is seen as a normal process, not an abnormal one. The birth lobby in Britain includes several organised groups and Well-Women Clinics centred on women's health care needs. Epidemiology is being recognised as essential to a full understanding of health and a necessary adjunct of medical care. Epidemiology is a branch of medical statistics which deals with the distribution and prevalence of diseases as influenced by the environment and behaviour; in trying to correlate presumed causal factors and the occurrence of illness, epidemiologists consider such variables as sex differences, marital status, occupation, social class, age, individual behaviour and environment as these bear heavily on distribution and prevalence of health and ill-health. This has been crucial for understanding, for example, which groups of women are most likely to be at risk of developing cervical cancer, a rising cause of fertility problems in women (Robinson, 1987).

All these examples show up that, on a most basic level, technological 'solutions' are not solutions. A great deal of reproductive health problems, including fertility problems and congenital conditions, can be eliminated with a women-centred approach to reproduction: with better primary health care, and changes in social and economic relations. The World Health organisation (WHO) reported that most infertility in the world is preventable (Diczfalusy, 1986). A symposium sponsored by WHO in October 1986, whose participants included women from many parts of the globe, concluded strongly:

> It should be acknowledged that the major hazard to the health of the woman and the newborn infant is poverty, and that, in the absence of concerted measures to promote social equity, only minimal changes in maternal and infant morality and morbidity can be expected. (*Women's World*, 1986, p. 36)

The starting point for reasserting a women-centred ethic is the reassertion that *women are our bodies* and *women are ourselves, autonomous*. Our Bodies, Ourselves is so obvious yet so revolutionary that it is a contemporary feminist statement. This is radical in a male-centred reality, where women's bodies have long been the site of reproductive control, where woman alone is anathema,[11] and where the term 'Man' still defines the generic human.

Mainstream ethical thought has been unable to contemplate women in relation to ourselves, that is women as women. I shall centre my critique on women as women, *decoupled* from men, to strike at the heart of the matter.

2

Status of the embryo

Feminists and many women who would not call themselves
feminists insist that discussions of pregnancy and childbirth are
discussions about women: women's lives, women's health, women's
right to control our own bodies. It is perfectly clear to us that the
health and well-being of offspring depends fundamentally on
women's health and well-being, which in turn depends on adequate
primary health care, nutrition, standards of living, and life-
respecting, woman-respecting social relations.

A woman-centred approach to pregnancy and childbirth places
priority on women's physical and emotional welfare, and the
principle that the welfare of mother and child are intertwined. The
Association of Radical Midwives in Britain, critical of the high-tech
approach to reproduction, stated in their 1986 Proposals for the
Future of Maternity Services 'that the mother is the central person
in the process of care' (ARM, 1986).

Recognising women as central subjects in human procreation has
been virtually unrecognised in the dominant 'public' debate on the
new reproductive technologies. Instead the status of the embryo/
fetus is the central subject of concern. In her enlightening article
'Fetalists and Feminists: They Are Not the Same' (1987), Janice
Raymond compares the fetal-centredness of two groups: (i)
anti-abortionists who oppose IVF, and (ii) IVF practitioners and
advocates of the new reproductive technologies. She names both
groups fetalists, for both in their distinctive ways centre their
concerns around the fetus, and both sorts of fetalists subordinate
women to their fetalist values.

Feminists who oppose the new reproductive technologies

(NRTs) are emphatically not political allies of anti-abortionists who oppose IVF/human embryo research. Feminist opposition to embryo research comes from concern with what it means for women. We can be both *for* women's right to abortion and *against* embryo research because we are concerned with women's reproductive freedom and health. An embryo or fetus is not a disembodied individual, as fetalists represent it.

In this chapter I concentrate on the other sort of fetalists: the reproductive technology advocates, to show how their fetus-centred reproductive practices and reproductive research is increasingly subordinating women to the fetus, and how this subordination oppresses women as a group.

I wish to make something very clear before going further. Later in the chapter I criticise the promotion by medical science and the state of eugenic abortion, that is abortion when a fetus is judged by medical tests to be 'abnormal' (for example, with Down's Syndrome). This is not an anti-abortionist stance. Rather, I wish to show up how medical science is being allowed to define the criteria for legal abortion in Western countries, while women are denied authority to make our own decisions about abortion. Later chapters further clarify the history of eugenic control of reproduction, for example through pre-natal screening and selective abortion. As our consciousness is raised about eugenics, we must all come to terms with what eugenic abortion means. But we can be perfectly clear, as Anne Finger (1984, p. 287) stated:

> No woman should be forced to bear a child, abled or disabled; and no progressive social movement should exploit an oppressed group to further its ends. We do not need, as Michelle Fine and Adrienne Asch point out, to list conditions – such as the presence of a fetus with a disability – under which abortion is acceptable. The right to abortion is not dependent on certain circumstances: it is our absolute and essential right to have control over our bodies.

Throughout this book I use both the terms 'embryo' and 'fetus', although they are actually the same topic. It would be possible simply to talk about fetuses throughout. However, I use 'embryo' for the earliest stages of development in a woman's pregnancy (e.g. for IVF embryos created with eggs removed from women), and the term 'fetus' for the time beyond (e.g. fetuses used in research which were acquired from women having abortions). Later in this chapter I discuss both words. My only reason in making a distinction is to represent the way both terms are being used by 'experts'.

The status of the embryo . . . devalues women

The status of the embryo is the central concern in the 'public' debate on IVF issues. The dominant ethical debate follows from a Western moral tradition which took the concept of 'formation' or 'animation' of the fetus from the language of Greek embryology. Greek philosophers and physicians imagined states of 'non-being' and 'being' in embryonic development, in concert with the question 'When does life begin?' Aristotle decided that male embryos 'form', or become 'being', at forty days gestation; females, imperfect males, 'form' at eighty days. The concept that life begins at some moment in development became part of Western intellectual thought and the basis for legal and moral sanctions imposed against abortion.

The question of the beginning of human life has been, and continues to be, a reflection of sexist thinking and practice. It has been and continues to be a criterion to judge and control women's reproductive behaviour. The question was first posed by intellectuals of a patriarchal society where women did not have autonomous political status. It has been perpetuated through the centuries by male intellectuals, philosophers, theologians, naturalists, judges.[1] Today, the question of embryonic life is the domain of biologists, too. The question did not come from women as pertinent to experience and knowledge of pregnancy.

The ancient Greek biology from which the original question of life arose is no longer scientifically credible. Today, for the most sophisticated scientists, the question 'When does life *begin*?' is inadequate, meaningless, absurd, unanswerable. For IVF pioneer Robert Edwards and IVF apologist Clifford Grobstein, life is a continuum, a process that proceeds through generations, not a moment in time. According to Edwards, the potentiality for life resides in women's unfertilised eggs and all its precurser cells. As an argument against 'life begins at fertilisation' he used the phenomenon of parthenogenesis, spontaneous division of an unfertilised egg cell which sometimes occurs in mammals (Edwards, 1974, p. 13). That is, he used it as an argument to present IVF practice as morally acceptable. The scientific rejection of pinpointing when life begins is not an act of humility, but fidelity to the biological 'facts' (what scientists know). IVF advocates use the 'biological evidence' that life-is-a-continuum ('evidence' gleaned from *in vitro* experiments with eggs and embryos in the first place) to counter claims of anti-abortionists who believe that human life begins at fertilisation and so oppose IVF.

However, biological facts do not speak for themselves. It does not follow that when scientists believe life-is-a-continuum, that they reject the 'status of the embryo' discussion and recognise women as the subject of procreation. For one, IVF advocates cannot completely reject the 'status of the embryo' even though the Greek biology from which the concept arose is no longer scientifically credible. For if scientists debating the ethics of embryo research reject the 'status of the embryo', they would be left with identifying women as the subject of IVF research. They would be left with having to debate the ethics of using women, not embryos, as experimental subjects. Scientists' defence of IVF must fit into the terms of the dominant, age-old ethical debate about embryos and reproduction. And that means coming to terms with the moral status of embryos/fetuses. From the beginning of the 'public' debate on the NRTs, medical scientists and the scientific establishment adapted the 'status of the embryo' to fit into the scientific context. It was necessary to deal with higher authorities such as government inquiries on their own moral terms.

Further, the understanding that life-is-a-continuum, when based on scientific knowledge, is so rarefied a concept that anti-abortionists can easily adapt the 'biological evidence' that life-is-a-continuum to argue against IVF/'human embryo' research, as did Stephen Browne in the *British Medical Journal* (1982). This may happen because modern scientific knowledge of reproduction is centred on the fetus, without consideration of women's experience of pregnancy and birth. Similarly, the anti-abortionists' world view does not consider women's subjectivity as whole human beings, but rather considers embryos' subjectivity as apart from women. Both anti-abortionist and IVF advocates arguing their opposing cases are preoccupied with an imaginary isolated cell-egg-embryo-fetus-newborn-Man, disconnected from a woman.

In short, the ancient question 'when does life begin?' is embryo-centred, a denial of women's subjectivity, and oppressive to women. But so is the contemporary *scientific* rejection of it. 'Life' from the male-centred scientific view perceives women in the role of a life-support system, not women as acting with nature in a conscious, human way during pregnancy and childbirth. As scientists working in the area of 'human reproduction' see it, indeed as one IVF practitioner put it, women are *biologically* no different from sheep or cows.[2]

What happens when IVF advocates try to mould the 'status of the embryo' to fit their needs to do 'human embryo' research (that is, research using women's eggs, wombs, bodies)? They are left with a moral paradox. On the one hand, they accept the special status of the embryo. On the other hand, the meaning of the embryo is changed when the sanctity of embryos is weighed against the interests of science in human embryo research, the 'needs' of reproducing couples (the needs *reproductive engineers* recognise) and eugenics (the science of trying to create 'better' offspring). This moral paradox and its link to the anti-abortionist agenda is mystified by IVF researchers. Australian IVF practitioner Carl Wood and two of his colleagues appeased right-to-lifers by saying that IVF is about preserving life, not destroying it (Walters and Singer, 1982, p. 38). Similarly, IVF doctor Jack Glatt (1982), in England, wrote that IVF is about creating life, not destroying it as in abortion. Yet the fact remains that many human embryos are inevitably discarded in IVF practice and human embryo research. By not mentioning that fact, IVF practitioners hope to convey that their concern for 'life' is praiseworthy whether their scientific interests are abstract (knowledge-acquiring) or centred on making babies.

When the abortion connection was recognised by British clinical geneticist and IVF advocate David Weatherall, women still came up short. To make a case for using genetic engineering methods in human embryo research, Weatherall argued, 'At first sight, it seems strange that a society which condones abortion for the most trivial social reasons should suddenly be so concerned about the human rights of embryos that it insists that they must be protected by law' (Weatherall, 1985, p. 190). For IVF advocate Weatherall women's reasons for seeking abortion are subsumed in the trivial. His message is that the immense benefit of genetic knowledge is most worthy.

A pregnant women is herself whole. Being woman-centred rather than embryo-centred, feminists reject the identification of a disembodied embryo. We reject defining the embryo as unconnected with the woman who carries it. We reject the identification of embryos as separate entities with separate interests whether by anti-abortionists, doctors, scientists, lawyers, politicians, ethicists or theologians. The conceptual split between woman and fetus comes from a Western, male, intellectual view of reproduction; it is enhanced by the new artificial reproduction technologies which *literally* split woman and embryo/fetus, a 'logical' progression from the mental split between woman and fetus in masculinist thinking. Research on artificial wombs is an extension of that split.

The mental split between woman and fetus is an imposition on women. Ultrasound scanning in pregnancy is one example of a technical invention being overused on women without adequate consideration of its possible long-term health risks. In medicine, ultrasound scanning is the use of high frequency sound waves to show visual outlines of internal body parts. In pregnancy it is used to observe the fetus inside the woman to determine gestational age, to look for abnormalities of the fetus and uterus, and to guide doctors performing other medical interventions on pregnant women (for instance during amniocentesis).

Ultrasound scanning is now widely used and often assumed to be safe, though no long-term studies on its effects have as yet been reported. Biologist Ruth Hubbard (1984) in the USA and social scientist Ann Oakley (1986) in Britain have both been critical of the use of ultrasound on large numbers of healthy pregnant women. Hubbard makes an analogy with the use of X-rays on pregnant women in the past, noting that it took twenty or thirty years before studies linked the use of pre-natal X-ray examinations to the production of leukemias and cancers. Looking at the 'discoveries' researchers have made about the gestating fetus using obstetrical ultrasound Ann Oakley notes, 'This hardly adds up to outstanding, original wisdom justifying the use of a potent technology. Any mother can tell you that fetuses don't always move in the same way, and that sometimes a healthy fetus doesn't move at all' (Oakley, 1986, p. 11). Also, the ultrasound picture is not necessarily welcome by a pregnant women. The fuzzy shape on a television screen can be deeply disconcerting, especially when women are not adequately prepared as to what to expect.[3] Still, enthusiasts of ultrasound claim that it helps a pregnant woman to bond with the fetus. Ann Oakley suggests that the pre-natal bonding phenomenon in ultrasound is a rediscovering-the-wheel activity of the most primitive kind. 'Mothers and newborns are in a relationship with one another before they meet on the ultrasound screen' (p. 12).

Technology sets the ethic, the ethic sets the technology

The fetus as a 'second patient' is being firmly esablished as a concept in obstetrics. In the USA Barbara Katz Rothman has written widely on the impact of pregnancy intervention technologies on women. She quotes the 1980 edition of a classic obstetrics textbook which states that the fetus has 'rightfully achieved the status of the second patient, a patient who usually faces much greater risk of morbidity and mortality than does the mother' (Rothman, 1984, pp. 25–6). In 1986, the medical journal *Fetal Therapy* appeared, advertised as the first to focus on the fetus as patient, with attention given to the moral and ethical issues of fetal intervention *in utero* [in a woman's body], the legal rights of the fetus, and the new concept of fetal personality, also known as fetal psychology. In the US, a number of institutions have appointed interdisciplinary committees of 'experts' to represent fetuses (Kolder *et al.*, 1987).

The medical status of the fetus *as distinct from the woman who is pregnant* is becoming a star criterion to judge a women's behaviour before, during, and after pregnancy. It is no longer only our sexuality or marital status which defines us as good woman–mothers; now, we must not smoke or drink or deny medical intervention when we are pregnant, or else we are not acting in the 'best interests of the fetus'. Meanwhile, obstetricians have authorised themselves to act against the wishes of the pregnant woman if necessary to 'protect' the interests of the fetus. They ponder a moral dilemma of their own construction, adopting the words of the legal profession: 'maternal versus fetal rights'. This is the language obstetricians are using to identify rights and interests of a fetus as sometimes in conflict with women's interests, desires, behaviour, and will. The perceived conflict between woman and fetus is similarly codified in other medical–legal terms such as fetal neglect, fetal rights, fetus-as-patient, and fetal therapy. (For examples see Bowes and Selgestad, 1985; Cinque, 1987; Elias and Annas, 1983; Fletcher, 1981; and Murray, 1985.) These concepts appear in medical textbooks and are taught to medical students. The ethic of serving the fetus as a distinct patient is in part due to these technologies. Obstetricians recognise that *their role as fetus-protectors comes from technology.*

For example, in the medical textbook *Principles of Medical Therapy* (1985), used in the top-ranking University of Pennsylvania Medical School, there appears a single-paged chapter entitled 'Maternal Versus Fetal Rights'. The authors, Leo R. Boler, Jr. and Norbert Gleicher, subscribe to the treatment of the fetus as a 'second patient once viability is achieved'. They take that to be twenty-four weeks, since, they explain, in the United States the fetus is recognised as having legal rights from twenty-four weeks gestational age.

Boler and Gleicher project the obstetrician's role as protector of the fetus against the passive or actively 'hostile' behaviour of the mother; and articulate the roots of their role in available technology:

> Thus, *a conflict between fetal and maternal rights* may arise that requires intervention by the treating physician and has in some instances reached the courts . . .
>
> Sometimes the intrauterine environment is *hostile* and will not, or not ideally, support life . . . Today, the obstetrician is able to assess this hostility of the intrauterine environment . . .
>
> The increasing sophistication of *fetal surveillance techniques* has inevitably led to medicolegal aspects of fetal treatments and procedures . . .
>
> Techniques of fetal monitoring . . . intrauterine fetal transfusions, intravenous administration of tocolytic agents and Caesarean section delivery represent only a few examples of *medical intervention in response to fetal indications that potentially may place the mother at risk.* In most cases, the mother is willing to accept the added risks of morbidity and mortality in the interest of her unborn infant. *However, when the mother is unwilling to accept such risks and refuses treatment, a precarious medicolegal situation arises.* (My emphasis)

These authors are setting up a situation where the life (mortality) of the woman is measured against that of the fetus. (Interestingly, one of them, Norbert Gleicher, is an editor-in-chief of *The Journal of In Vitro Fertilisation and Embryo Transfer*, which first appeared in 1984).

These fetal-centred issues were discussed at a seminar in the US held by obstetricians on the 'ethical dilemma [which] arises when a pregnant woman refuses treatment that would benefit her fetus'. A report of the meeting stated: 'Dr Chervenak believes that a woman in labour who refuses to have a Caesarean section when her fetus shows signs of distress may not be thinking rationally because of pain and fear of labour. The risk of preventable ischemic brain damage or fetal death in this situation overrides the obstetrician's obligation to respect maternal autonomy.' Dr Chervenak was quoted: 'If persuasion failed, I would be prepared to restrain the mother and do the Caesarean section because of an overwhelming obligation to protect fetal well-being' (Koch, 1985).

Legal sanctions imposed against abortion embody this thinking. They pre-date the phrase 'maternal versus fetal rights', but similarly identify a distinct fetus that requires protection from women and abortionists. The medical profession acts as the agent of the state in providing that protection. One accepted 'medical' reason for abortion is if pre-natal screening shows that the fetus is 'abnormal'. Selective abortion of 'abnormal' fetuses is often called therapeutic abortion or negative eugenics, decreasing the propagation of certain types of offspring. 'Abnormal' fetuses are not as protected by the medical profession as are 'healthy' fetuses. Many Western countries (but not all, Ireland is an obvious exception) hold a policy of negative eugenics, encouraging abortion of fetuses which are identified 'abnormal' by genetic screening technology (what doctors can do).

Going a step further, the medical profession's expanded role today as protectors of the fetus is based on their capabilities and knowledge due to so-called advances in 'fetology' (a relatively new discipline). Medical knowledge about conception and pregnancy, brought to us with the aid of intervention technologies such as ultrasound for fetal monitoring, has helped create the basis for legal action against women in the name of 'protection of the unborn child'. However, as in abortion, the medical profession has been generally reluctant to protect the life of a 'deformed' fetus with medical interventions (Kaufmann and Williams, 1985).

'Fetal neglect' action has been taken against pregnant women, birthing women, and women after the birth of a child. Pregnant women have been jailed in the USA to prevent their drinking alcohol when doctors identified a risk of 'fetal alcohol syndrome'. In another instance, a doctor obtained a court order to give an intrauterine blood transfusion against the objections of the pregnant woman, who had refused on religious grounds. Also in the USA, there have been a number of cases in which doctors obtained court orders to force birthing women to undergo Caesarean sections. A woman in California was brought to trial for taking drugs during pregnancy. In another case, a women was arrested for failing to go to the hospital soon after she began haemorrhaging when pregnant; her baby subsequently died and the blame was put on her lack of action. In 1986, in Britain, five Law Lords unanimously upheld the right of magistrates to take a newborn baby away from her mother who was addicted to heroin during pregnancy. The baby was removed from the mother's care immediately after the birth and given to foster parents with the intention that adoptive parents would eventually be found. The court decision was not based on the ability of the mother to care for the child after the birth, but on her behaviour during pregnancy. The Law Lords set a precedent for the protection of fetuses under already existing laws for the protection of children; Britain has no official legal recognition of fetal rights (yet). Still, the decision was a *de facto* fetal neglect ruling. (These cases are cited in Koch, 1985; Dean, 1986; Boler and Gleicher, 1985; Rothman, 1984; *Breaking Chains*, 1986.)

In the USA, there is official legal recognition of fetal rights. In 1987, *The New England Journal of Medicine* published the results of a national survey investigating court-ordered obstetrical interventions on pregnant women who had refused to undergo a procedure ordered by the doctor. As the authors of the survey wrote, 'Proponents of forced treatment have focused on the legal status of the fetus.' The results are so obviously telling that I quote extensively from the abstract:

Court orders have been obtained for Caesarean sections in 11 states, for hospital detentions in 2 states, and for intrauterine transfusions in 1 state. Among 21 cases in which court orders were sought, the orders were obtained in 86 per cent; in 88 per cent of those cases, the orders were received within six hours. Eighty-one percent of the woman involved were black, Asian, or Hispanic, 44 per cent were unmarried, and 24 per cent did not speak English as their primary language. All the women were treated in a teaching-hospital clinic or were receiving public assistance. No important maternal morbidity or mortality was reported. Forty-six percent of the heads of fellowship programmes in maternal–fetal medicine thought that women who refused medical advice and thereby endangered the life of the fetus should be detained. Forty-seven percent supported court orders for procedures such as intrauterine transfusions. (Kolder *et al.*, (1987, p. 1192)

It is not surprising that the most vulnerable women in the population are the first to have these procedures forced on them. It is not surprising that these occurrences are taking place in prestigious teaching hospitals. It is horrifying that so many specialist doctors in obstetrics approve of these tactics. The three authors of the survey are two obstetricians, Veronika Kolder and Michael Parsons, and a civil rights lawyer, Janet Gallagher. They see this trend as a growing problem across the USA. None of the women 'was deemed incompetent', they note. The women's refusals were based on reasons such as religious belief or disagreement with the doctor's judgement. They make an important point that 'Uncertainty is intrinsic to medical judgement' and they cite several cases where the medical judgement for Caesarean section was wrong.

Medical control of women spreads to other areas of women's pregnancy. In Wisconsin, a pregnant teenager has been held in secure detention for the sake of the fetus because she 'tended to be "on the run" ' (Ibid., p. 1195). If US courts choose to further uphold the 'rights' of fetuses, laws restricting the liberties of all women of childbearing age would be needed. Janet Gallagher believes that the legal precedents already established in the US may lead to a 'police state for women' (*Scientific American*, 1987).

Fetus-directed technology incorporates the medically defined reality and 'ethic', to the detriment of women. The meaning of the fetus-*in-utero* hinges on technological capabilities which embody the fetalist values of their inventors. One of the roots of this fetal-centred medical stance comes from scientific experiments on 'artificial wombs', experiments on keeping fetuses and premature babies alive in laboratories. *In vitro* experiments with fetuses and placentae paved the way for the 'isolated fetus', disembodied from the mother. By the early 1970s, British physiologists were talking about the fetus and placenta as a 'functional metabolic unit', and the almost 'independent' role of the placenta in maintaining pregnancy (Macnaughton, 1973).

Research scientists refined their concepts of the 'maternal–fetal relationship' from their laboratory experiments with 'isolated fetuses'. In 1977, Professor Robert McCance outlined the change in the researcher's consciousness of the relationship between woman and fetus. He wrote that the 'old' concept from the late 1960s was that the fetus and mother live in 'untroubled symbiosis'. He suggested that if contemporary scientific knowledge was accepted, then that concept would 'have to go and be replaced by the thought that they are really rubbing along together in a state of armed neutrality' (McCance, 1977, p. 154, references removed). Neither assessment comes from women's diverse experiences of pregnancy. They are judgements coming from scientists working on 'isolated fetuses' who then decided in one decade that women are passive receptacles, and then in another decade that we are antagonists.

The point that reproductive technology sets the ethic of the fetus becomes crystal clear if we look at the political meaning of neonatal technology. This refers to the care of very premature babies, born before the age of 'viability', the 'date from which a fetus could be regarded as capable of being born alive' (Peel, 1979). There have been several attempts to restrict Britain's Abortion Act 1967 due to a changing definition of 'viability' based on medical capabilities in neonatal technology. In 1979, the then president of the Royal College of Obstetricians and Gynaecologists (RCOG), Sir John Peel, wrote a letter to the *British Medical Journal* supporting one such attempt, the Corrie Abortion Amendment Bill. The amendment, which the British Medical Association (BMA) did not support, would have shortened the upper time limit for abortion from twenty-eight weeks to twenty weeks. Peel wrote that, due to medical advances in neonatal technology, fetuses as young as twenty weeks could be kept alive and so the meaning of viability has changed. He added that this twenty-week viability figure should be kept under constant review in the light of increased developments in neonatal care (Ibid.).

Women's sensuous reproduction is lost in this *medical* meaning of 'viability'. After all, each pregnancy is unique, and why should pregnancy be defined with respect to the super-technology necessary to maintain 20-week-old fetuses? The medical concept of viability based on technology (what doctor's can do) upholds the power of the state and medical profession and warrants further restrictions on women. Although a twenty-eight-week upper time limit is still (in 1987) the law in Britain, most private clinics and charity trusts which offer abortion services have agreed to maintain a twenty-four week upper limit according to the Department of Health and Social Security's wishes. Lowering the upper time limit to twenty weeks would result in a similar situation, with the actual time limit being eighteen weeks.[4] As one doctor who criticised Peel's endorsement of the Corrie Abortion Amendment Bill pointed out, such a bill would have implicated more women than the few who would seek a late-term abortion. With its deft wording, the bill would have deprived 70 000 women each year of access to legal abortion in Britain (Huntingford, 1979). The bill did not pass.

In 1985, the RCOG issued a report of a working party which they set up, including representation from the BMA, the Royal College of Midwives, the British Paediatric Association, and the Royal College of General Practitioners (RCOG *et al.*, 1985). The report recommends that the Abortion Act 1967 be amended by changing the upper time limit from twenty-eight weeks to twenty-four weeks due to advances in neonatal technology. Now this is interesting in light of the 1979 letter from Peel which called for a twenty-week upper limit due to advances in technology. Why was technology so advanced in 1979 to warrant a twenty-week upper limit, while in 1985 a twenty-four-week upper limit was considered sufficient? The report (p. 15) explained that the decision was a 'balance between conflicting interests', that is, capabilities in neonatal technology and the shortcomings of pre-natal screening technology. They note that the 'majority of fetuses' capable of surviving would be protected, while 'women with currently acceptable reasons for legal abortion would still have time to obtain one'. What they meant by 'acceptable reasons for legal abortion' was eugenic abortion of fetuses judged abnormal by amniocentesis. Genetic screening technology – amniocentesis – was the limiting factor. The extra two weeks gives women time to have amniocentesis and, if warranted, choose an abortion for the negative eugenic reasons the state and medical profession allow.

This attempt at limiting abortion options for women, *initiated by the medical profession*, not by politicians, lawyers or religious groups, follows from their assessment of technology.[5] This can change again with technology, of course. Chorionic villi sampling (CVS), a relatively new pre-natal screening method, allows genetic testing as early as eight-weeks into pregnancy. If the CVS method becomes widely accepted in Britain, the RCOG can readapt the meaning of viability without consideration of the time gap presented by amniocentesis. Further into the future, there is the implication of the artificial womb. Robert Edwards pointed out in 1974 that almost one-half of pregnancy can be maintained outside the women's body, since IVF embryos could be kept alive for six days, mid-term abortuses can be maintained under laboratory conditions for a few hours or days, and premature human babies can be 'incubated' from twenty-four weeks (Edwards, 1974, p. 7). As research on human embryos and fetuses forges ahead, more stages of pregnancy will be able to be maintained by scientists. With a few turns of the technological screws, abortion should cease to be an option altogether.

The fetus has acquired an independent medical identity in part due to growing capabilities in reproductive technology. IVF technology takes the split between woman and fetus further. IVF practitioners create a literal split between woman and embryo, and then wax philosophical about it. Writing on the topic of frozen embryos in the esteemed *New England Journal of Medicine*, Clifford Grobstein and co-authors state that 'embryo survival and maternal interest are not opposed [as in abortion], since the embryo's development, at least theoretically, can continue in a uterus other than that of the genetic mother' (Grobstein *et al.*, 1985, p. 1586). They added that the ability to freeze human embryos extends the autonomy and independence of the embryo, disconnecting it from the mother's body indefinitely. For them, the woman disappears altogether, and a *Brave New World* scenario appears. They write: 'In effect, freezing not only disconnects an embryo from its production cycle in the donor [woman] but greatly facilitates transfer to nondonors [women who might receive the thawed embryo]' (p. 1585). Production cycle in the donor?

The authors also discuss the possibilities of using frozen embryos for embryo adoption, surrogacy, family planning for fertile couples who might choose to freeze a few IVF embryos and then be sterilised, and even 'transfers over long distances, as might be useful in extraterrestrial colonization'. Remember, this is the prestigious *New England Journal of Medicine*, not pop-science-digest. Women's bodies are needed for their earthly social activities and their colonial adventures. Women would thus be under the control of social engineers from adoption agencies to psychologists to medical professionals to IVF scientists, not to mention space scientists.

In another disgraceful episode in embryo ethics, in 1986 an Australian IVF team at Flinders Medical Centre in Adelaide, South Australia, published their technique for freezing women's eggs. This has been a more difficult feat than freezing embryos. This development was portrayed in the media as being of great benefit because now the moral problems of freezing embryos, of spare embryos and of 'wastage' of embryos was 'solved' (*New Scientist*, 1986a; Newsome, 1986). Women's bodies, where eggs and embryos come from, are not a presence in this kind of logic. Women go through exactly the same invasive drug and surgical procedures whether it is the egg that is frozen or the embryo that is frozen. Where is the concern for women, who are used for developing both techniques for freezing eggs and freezing embryos?

Embryo protection . . . disinherits women

In the wake of the British Warnock Report's endorsement of human embryo research, arch-conservative Member of Parliament Enoch Powell introduced an embryo protection bill in November 1984 called the Unborn Children (Protection) Bill. The Powell bill would have banned human embryo research. In effect, it would have stopped the use of IVF in clinical practice as well. Powell is avidly anti-abortion and anti-divorce. His ban on embryo research stems from his concern over the humanity of embryos, not the humanity of women.

The Conservative Government did not support Powell's bill (the government presumably supports Warnock Report recommendations and so is pro-embryo research). But Powell did receive a great deal of support in Parliament across party political lines. The bill might have passed, but it was eventually 'talked out' in a procedural manoeuvre without a vote. If it had passed, it would have opened the door to an anti-abortionist challenge of legal abortion. The bill reappeared twice as the Hargreaves bill.

Reacting to the threat of the Powell bill a lobby group called Progress was formed to promote IVF and human embryo research. Many scientists, politicians and women's rights activists are involved in the Progress lobby. The 'progress' it refers to is scientific progress, and the 'need' for scientists to pursue human embryo research for all sorts of reproductive engineering reasons. The literature Progress circulates aims to convince the public of the worth of the scientific pursuit of IVF/'human embryo' research. Progress is not a campaign to decriminalise abortion, and it was not formed as a women's rights lobby. However, many women involved believe Progress is necessary for stemming the right-wing repressive tide of anti-abortionists. Of course, fighting against embryo protection bills such as the offensive Powell and Hargreaves bills is necessary, for they will be used to further erode women's rights in the name of embryo protection. But we do not have to accept the terms of a lobby committed to ensuring the continuation of research on using women's body parts: eggs and *in vitro* embryos. Why settle for an either/or situation? Criticising groups promoting 'human embryo' research such as Progress does not mean aligning with Powell's right. Neither point of view is women-centred. Powell and company want to 'protect' embryos and families (control women's reproductive role within a patriarchal family). But resisting anti-abortionists and embryo protection bills by aligning with IVF advocates also marginalises women. It means walking a tightrope in the 'status of the embryo' game, accepting the split between an embryo and woman by saying women's rights to abortion *and* medical scientists rights to do 'embryo research' (so-called progress) override 'protection of the embryo'. Why accept the language of fetalists? As Janice Raymond (1987) points out, raising the status of women is necessary to raise the status of motherhood; but raising the status of women is not on the fetalist agenda: neither the anti-technology anti-abortion agenda nor the pro-technology pro-embryo research agenda.

Embryo protection bills are not only the tactic of anti-abortionists. A West German Embryo Protection Bill was proposed in 1986 by the Minister of Justice, a liberal and not an anti-abortionist. Paragraph 1 of the bill contains the possibility of the law taking criminal action against pregnant women who knowingly damage a fetus, for example by taking drugs. The bill is being promoted as 'strict' regulation on reproductive technologies, again showing up the inability of those in power to think about protection of *women* on whom these technologies are used, and their continual attempts at restricting women's reproductive autonomy in the name of the fetus at any chance they get.

Introducing the pre-embryo or what's in a name?

Consider the world from the fetalist's perspective. Consider the word 'embryo' and its companion term 'fetus'. When does an embryo become a fetus? The word 'embryo' comes from the Greek; 'fetus', from the Latin. In common usage, 'fetus' refers to the gestating embryo after a certain time in development. In scientific parlance, usage varies considerably. The distinction between embryo and fetus is not, and never has been, fixed. Usage varies depending on the context, individual preference, or convention.

In Britain, the Council for Science and Society, reporting on ethical considerations of IVF in 1984, employed what they considered common usage. The human embryo was defined as the organism at early stages of development before recognisable human features are formed, at about eight weeks' gestation. While the fetus was defined as the developing human organism from eight weeks onward, after recognisable human features are formed. This is in agreement with some dictionaries of biology which make a distinction between embryo and fetus, but not all. (Of course, it depends on the meaning of 'recognisable'.) The British Warnock Inquiry adopted the term 'embryo' to mean the developing organism starting at fertilisation.

Scientists sometimes recognise this distinction between embryo and fetus, but sometimes do not. The word fetus does not appear in the 1985 edition of the *Oxford Dictionary of Natural History*, but the word embryo does. On the other hand, a collection of scientific articles entitled *The Mammalian Fetus In Vitro* (1973) takes the fetus (including the human fetus) to be the organism from implantation onwards. In the textbook, *Conception in the Human Female* (1980), Robert Edwards uses the word embryo to designate the organism during the early stages of development up to implantation; while the fetus is the human organism at and after implantation, from five days onward. For researchers like Edwards, under the general category 'embryo' are several other terms to designate different stages in development. The embryo may be identified as a zygote, a morula, a blastocyst, and so on.

Reconsider the embryo. The 'public' ethical debate over IVF prompted a new pertinent question. When does an embryo become an embryo?

The Warnock Report (1984) recommended allowing 'human embryo research' up to fourteen days after fertilisation *in vitro*.[6] The chosen fourteen-day limit was only one of many criteria suggested to the Warnock Committee by doctors and scientists. The Warnock decision is an arbitrary cut-off, as all agree. The 'scientific basis' of a fourteen-day limit is no more significant, scientifically speaking, than another. For example, some IVF 'experts' suggest that scientists should be granted use of six-week-old human embryos for research. Both a fourteen-day limit and a six-week limit have arguable scientific rationales.

Underlying the fourteen-day limit are a variety of scientific explanations that were put forward by 'experts' giving evidence to government committes. One scientist explained to the US Ethics Advisory Board that 'developmental individuality' is not established at fertilisation. The evidence scientists give for this is that at early stages in development the embryo may split into twins; also, two or more *in vitro* embryos can be fused together to form one embryo. Thus unique individuality is said to be established when the embryo can no longer become more or less than one, at about two weeks. A second explanation for choosing a fourteen-day limit stresses another way of looking at the same thing: at about two weeks, differentiation begins, where changes in cells specialise them into specific kinds of tissue and organs. Cell differentiation is directed by genetic mechanisms. In other words, this scientific explanation of individuality is bound up in '*genetic* identity' of the individual embryo. Of course, the unspoken presumption in each of these rationales is that scientific knowledge now defines human individuality. Much of this scientific knowledge came from *in vitro* experiments with embryos in the first place.

Similarly, underlying a six-week upper limit on research is a scientific rationale. It is slightly before the stage in development at which the embryo becomes 'sentient', that is, when it can react to stimuli. According to scientific wisdom, the embryo could feel pain by this stage. Thus, the six-week time limit appears relatively humane, since scientists tell us the embryo cannot feel pain until about the seventh or eighth week. Women, of course, feel pain throughout many of the IVF procedures preceding the creation of the research embryo. And of course, the scientific assessment could be wrong, since scientific knowledge about cells and the nature of fetal pain is limited. The Council for Science and Society in Britain recommended a six-week limit in their 1984 report drawn up by nine doctors and scientists under the chair of theologian Professor Gordon Dunstan.[7] In the US, the Ethics Advisory Board hearings considered this longer limit as well, although they finally recommended a fourteen-day limit in their 1979 report.

Only *after* the fourteen-day limit on human embryo research became the rule in Britain because of the Warnock Committee decision, and only *after* the threat of Enoch Powell's parliamentary bill banning *all* IVF/embryo research, did scientists in Britain publicly promote a scientific explanation for the fourteen-day limit. It was obviously an appeal to gain public support for human embryo research, as I will explain.

The Warnock Report recommended in 1984 that the British Government endorse IVF and human embryo research up to fourteen days and that they create a statutory licensing authority to oversee it. But the government repeatedly postponed acting on these sensitive issues (government sponsored legislation is possible in 1988). Prompted by the threat of the Powell bill, the MRC and RCOG established the Voluntary Licensing Authority (VLA) in early 1985 to oversee IVF practice and human embryo research along the lines the Warnock Report recommended. One of the VLA's first *self-assigned* tasks was to define what an embryo is.

Soon after the establishment of the VLA was announced, former President of the Royal Society Sir Andrew Huxley explained the fourteen-day limit in the popular magazine *New Scientist*. Huxley explained that for the first two weeks after fertilisation the cells of the growing conceptus are engaged in life-support work, for instance, making cells that will become placenta; thus only a few per cent of the cells become the 'embryo proper'. At fifteen or sixteen days the primitive streak appears where the 'definitive embryo' begins to form (Huxley, 1985). By his logic, the moral status of the embryo is set by the meaning embryologists give to embryos, based on *their* present-day knowledge, what they assess as significant, and just as importantly, on their presumption that the 'few per cent' of cells which are considered the presursor cells of the 'embryo proper' are *not* significant.

Two months after Huxley's article appeared the VLA introduced a brand new word 'pre-embryo' (Turney, 1985). A pre-embryo, we are told, is the group of cells growing from a fertilised human egg until the time the first signs of individual development appear, at about two weeks after fertilisation. This new term exactly categorises the embryo allowed for research purposes. Where did it come from? It was coined by a lay member of the VLA in preference to other terms they were considering to serve the same purpose such as conceptus, zygote, and pro-embryo.[8] These three terms are biological terms, and appear in biological dictionaries, but none of them is used in the strict sense for which the VLA was going to use them.

Embryologist and member of the Warnock Committee Anne McLaren subsequently wrote an article for *New Scientist* repeating Huxley's explanation about the fourteen-day limit on embryo research, but this time introducing the word pre-embryo. She did not make clear in this article that this was a newly coined term.

The term pre-embryo does not clarify the issues, as McLaren had offered; it obscures them. And it is manipulative. to start calling the early embryo a pre-embryo at this stage is a cheat. It erases the history of the decision about the fourteen-day limit. It makes it appear to those not familiar with that history as if the decision was inevitable, as if 'embryos' have never really existed until fourteen days after fertilisation *in vitro*.

The coining of the term pre-embryo was a political act. The 'pre-embryo' explanation from scientists has been tailored from the scientific 'facts' to accommodate the fourteen-day time limit, not vice-versa. The word pre-embryo was invented for the purpose of human embryo research. It was taken up by the media, by scientific journals, by the medical and science bodies formalising their regulations on IVF/human embryo research, and by the lobby group Progress whose aim is to promote 'human embryo' research through the public understanding of the scientific issues. The term was quickly picked up for usage in the journal *Nature* (Clarke, 1986). However, a former editor of *Nature*, David Davies (1986), criticised his colleagues for using the term instead of debating the issue directly, and Mary Warnock has never mentioned the term in public as far as I know. The term is being used by the American Fertility Society in the USA and by some 'human embryo' research advocates in Australia.

Interestingly, in May 1987, an editorial in *Nature* (p. 87) said the word pre-embryo was a 'cop-out', and called for a ban on using it. They did not mention that the word graced their own pages as acceptable usage sixteen months earlier.

IVF knowledge of embryos, fetuses and now 'pre-embryos' is yet another example of the power of medicine and science over women's fertility. IVF 'experts' are setting themselves up as authorities on making moral judgements about tampering with women's bodies and calling it moral judgements about embryos and pre-embryos. They have yet to address the ethics of using women's bodies in the scientific quest for 'knowledge' about women's reproduction.

The fourteen-day limit is not the last word in 'human embryo research'. Many IVF researchers in Britain 'do not want this to become an immovable obstacle for research on older embryos' (Connor, 1985). It is obvious that one reason the fourteen-day limit is so far acceptable to medical scientists is because researchers could not then keep human embryos alive *in vitro* past that limit anyway; someday they may be able to grow embryos past fourteen days, and many researchers look forward to the kinds of experiments they might then carry out. Why think of an end-point for embryo research, while mid-term fetuses acquired from women having abortions have been used for experimentation since the 1950s?[9]

Mary Warnock also implied that a longer time limit was possible at a lecture on Toleration, in 1987, in York. She suggested that perhaps the criterion that a fetus feels pain could be used by law-makers in deciding the limits of embryo research. This implies a six-week limit. *Any* such criterion about the protection of embryos (not women) set down in law works against women, the most obvious effect is that it would open the door to anti-abortionists wishing to limit legal abortion, and the possibility of 'fetal neglect' action being taken against pregnant women and perhaps any woman of childbearing age. Again, this is the dilemma for women within a fetalist ethic. If there is no statutory time limit on embryo/fetus research, then scientists may have uncontrolled access to women's bodies for experimentation. If there is a legal time limit placed on embryo research, then women are left to fight against losing our rights and autonomy to the legal status of embryos.

The term 'status of the embryo' is about the power of men, of the state, and of medicine and science over women. The state and medical scientists – the keepers of ideology and the makers of technology – collude to construct a meaning of the embryo as 'natural', hiding its misogynist history. They construct the image of the embryo as essential, central to the ethics and the technology.

The myth of the unencumbered, free-floating embryo, and the identification of IVF embryos as the subject of reproduction are tricks against women. The use of the 'biological facts' to define the embryo protects medical scientists and their interests. This should be obvious since medicine and science has defined the terrain – embryos, pre-embryos, isolated fetuses – from their own point of view in the first place. Their fetal-centred point of view, their fetal-centred technology, and their authority as 'experts' on reproduction place women's physical bodies at the service of fetus-oriented medical scientists. The women's health movement wants to see the orientation of medical science changed to consider women as the central subject of pregnancy.

3

IVF on women

'Test-tube' babies are not grown in test tubes as the name might imply. Louise Brown and the many hundreds of 'test-tube' babies around the world were conceived by IVF (*in vitro* fertilisation), where women's eggs are removed from our ovaries and fertilised in a laboratory dish with men's sperm. If a normal looking embryo results, it is inserted into the woman's womb. The embryo insertion procedure is called embryo replacement or embryo transfer.

Several variations of the basic IVF protocol exist. For example in GIFT, gamete intrafallopian transfer, the woman's egg is removed but the fertilisation is not destined to occur in the laboratory dish. The removed and matured egg and sperm are inserted into the woman's fallopian tube where hopefully fertilisation will take place. In another procedure used in France, Intra-Vaginal Culture and Embryo Transfer (IVCET), eggs are removed from the woman, placed with sperm in one or more boxes, and then placed into her vagina 'instead of an incubator' (Laborie, 1987). Another IVF variation is 'egg donation', where a woman donates one or more of her eggs to another woman (couple) in an IVF programme. Removal of women's eggs and keeping them alive under laboratory conditions is the key to a variety of IVF related clinical procedures, and it is a precondition for research on *in vitro* human embryos, for genetic selection of early embryos, and for future prospects in genetic engineering ('genetic therapy') of early embryos.

Below I describe the bare bones of the basic IVF protocol used for clinical treatment of fertility problems.[1]

Evaluation

Before a woman is accepted into an IVF programme she is evaluated medically and socially. As a rule, in Britain, as in most countries, only heterosexual couples living together in 'stable' relationships are eligible. Marital stability and ability to cope with the procedures is evaluated by the IVF practitioners and their team. Some IVF teams include psychologists who conduct the social evaluation. Certain types of infertility are considered treatable by IVF, such as blocked tubes, male subfertility and 'unexplained' infertility (this is a medical category).

The reasons for using IVF on women, the 'medical indications', are growing, and this has been the case with other medical technologies, such as Caesarean section and pre-natal screening. IVF was first recommended as a last resort treatment for women who could not conceive because of blocked tubes. Now IVF is considered an acceptable treatment for several, but not all, kinds of female fertility problems. With 'egg donation' IVF is indicated for those who cannot produce eggs, and for women who are 'carriers' of genetic disease. IVF is also being used as a treatment for subfertility in men, even if the woman herself is fertile, as fertilisation may be forced in a laboratory dish. The risk of damage from manipulations into a woman's healthy internal organs – a major known cause of infertility – is hardly mentioned when these uses of IVF are put forward.

If a couple's fertility problems fit into the indications for IVF, the woman often undergoes a preliminary procedure, called laparoscopy (described below), to evaluate the condition of her ovaries.

Fertility management

Egg retrieval is described by medical scientists both as complicated and experimental, and as straightforward and routine. How can it be both? It entails physical and biochemical manipulation of women's bodies. Sometimes the IVF practitioner relies on a woman's 'spontaneous' menstrual cycle for the collection of a single ripe egg. Usually, however, the overian cycle is artifically *stimulated* and *controlled* with fertility drugs. These might be naturally occurring hormones, non-hormonal drugs, or synthetic hormone analogues chemically related (but not identical) to naturally occurring hormones. These drugs are not specific to IVF, but are used in a variety of applications on women as fertility therapies. Ovulation, menstruation and pregnancy involve an elaborate sequence of interactions among hormones from the anterior pituitary gland, the hypothalamas, the ovaries, and the adrenal cortex. Fertility management drugs disrupt the women's own hormonal interplay.[2]

Stimulation of women's ovaries with drugs so that they produce many eggs per cycle, instead of the usual one egg, is called superovulation or hyperovulation. At first, we heard that four or six or eights eggs were being extracted from women's ovaries using these methods. Then came reports of fourteen and seventeen.

For an example of one often-used regimen, the fertility drug clomiphene citrate and/or the hormone HMG (human menopausal gonadotropin) are administered to stimulate the woman's ovaries to produce multiple eggs. Clomiphene citrate is a synthetic estrogen (hormone) used to induce ovulation. It has many adverse effects, including enlargement of the ovaries, and in some cases contributes to fertility problems by adversely effecting the post-ovulatory phase of a woman's menstrual cycle. HMG is a commercial preparation of two hormones, FSH and LH (follicle stimulating hormone and luteinising hormone). Its purpose is to bypass the hypothalamus and pituitary gland to stimulate the ovaries and induce ovulation. It is extremely powerful and carries risks of overstimulation and enlargement of the ovaries. It is also extremely expensive. FSH and LH are naturally occurring menstrual cycle hormones; both are secreted by the anterior pituitary gland, and are necessary for the proper functioning of the ovaries and other reproductive processes. HMG is acquired from the urine of newly menopausal women.

Timing of ovulation may be controlled by other drugs. For example, an injection of HCG (human chorionic gonadotropin) may be administered to trigger ovulation as part of an HMG or clomiphene citrate regimen. The IVF practitioner can thus predict the timing of ovulation for egg retrieval. Controlling the timing of ovulation is considered necessary, not least for the convenience of the surgeon and hospital staff. IVF practitioners in Britain, France and Australia admit this (see Laborie, 1987; Trounson and Conti, 1982; Fleming *et al.*, 1985). HCG is a naturally occurring menstrual cycle hormone which induces egg maturation and ovulation; it is acquired from the urine of pregnant women.

Several permutations of stimulation and control of the woman's menstrual cycle are used by IVF practitioners. Which hormones a woman is given, which protocol the IVF practitioner follows, whether the women's cycle is stimulated or controlled or both depends on the particular IVF team.

Some women are left to a 'natural cycle', one reason being in order that the success rate of embryo implantation may be compared with women whose cycles are controlled and stimulated. The problem for IVF practitioners is that the drugs seem to hinder the implantation of the inserted IVF embryo, and thus the 'success rate' of their IVF programmes. As the efficacy of the various regimens is in question, IVF practitioners continue to experiment with different kinds of drugs, and carry out studies comparing one regimen with another.

Some of the drugs being used on IVF programmes are chemically related to known carcinogens (Direcks, 1987), and fertility drugs are associated with high rates of miscarriage. The possible risks to women of ovarian cysts and other damage to the ovaries and menstrual cycle from IVF manipulation is infrequently mentioned by IVF practitioners, and only in the bowels of the medical literature.

Throughout this first phase of IVF, the woman's fertility is monitored daily, eventually twice daily, with urine tests and/or blood tests to measure hormone levels in order to pinpoint the time of ovulation. As the time of ovulation nears, ultrasound is used to measure the size (maturity) of the follicles containing developing eggs. The woman on IVF must be available and fully committed. Christine Crowe reports that women she spoke to on IVF programmes in Australia explained that the commitment often entails relocating and putting off life plans for the duration of the programme (Crowe, 1987a).

It is important to mention here, since I do not expand on it elsewhere, the mutually obliging relationship between commercial interests and IVF interests. Medical supply companies gain from the demand for and sale of testing kits for urine and blood analysis, specialised IVF equipment, culture media, and so on. Pharmaceutical companies develop and supply the hormone drugs, such as clomiphene citrate as Clomid from Merrell, HMG as Pergonal from Serono, HCG as Pregnyl from Organon, FSH as Metrodin from Serono, and an analogue of LHRH (luteinising hormone releasing hormone) called Buserelin from Hoechst. These companies encourage researchers by donating drugs for clinical research projects. The researchers in turn acquire expensive and sometime novel drugs, and they duly acknowledge the support of the companies and corporations. Organon and Serono provided the major financial backing for the second conference of the medical/scientific European Society of Human Reproduction and Embryology (ESHRE) in 1986, and have promised to continue that support (Burfoot, 1987). ESHRE was born out of the IVF era; one of its founders is IVF pioneer Robert Edwards.

Egg retrieval

Eggs are usually removed from women's ovaries when ripe but before they leave the follicles. Laparoscopy is the major procedure used for collection of ripe eggs, or 'harvesting' eggs as the medical literature sometimes states. It was perfected by the British IVF pioneer Patrick Steptoe. Laparoscopic egg retrieval is a surgical technique requiring general anaesthesia and distension of the woman's abdomen with a carbon dioxide gas mixture. To remove eggs, the doctor makes three incisions below the woman's navel through which instruments are inserted. The laparoscope is a light guide allowing observation of the ovaries; a pair of forceps is used to grasp and rotate the ovary; and a suction device is used to pull out ripe eggs from their follicles. Sometimes it works, sometimes the doctor fails to remove the ripe eggs.

Another egg retrieval technique invented for IVF is called TUDOR, Trans Vaginal Ultrasound Directed Oocyte Recovery, developed in Sweden, Denmark and Austria. This method's purported advantage over laparoscopy is that it does not require general anaesthesia and is cheaper to use. However, as Renate Klein (1986) points out, it is highly painful for the woman, and many doctors have returned to using general anaesthesia or medications to numb the pain. Also, there are other problems and harmful effects. The woman's bladder is emptied with a catheter and refilled with saline solution. A needle for pulling out mature eggs is inserted through her vagina and into the bladder and towards the ovary. An ultrasound scan guides the doctor moving the needle around. Fewer eggs are gleaned from TUDOR, since the eggs are more difficult to grasp than in laparoscopy; and damage to the bladder is a dangerous risk. As Klein writes: 'The method which was hailed as a major technological advance does not seem to be too promising, after all.' (In yet another method of egg retrieval, a long needle is inserted through the woman's abdomen as an ultrasound scan guides the doctor.)

Semen collection

About two hours before egg retrieval, semen is collected from the male partner of the woman. He masturbates into a sterile cup. Some IVF clinics stock pornographic magazines for the man's use. The collected semen is washed and concentrated.

Fertilisation *in vitro*

If the IVF practitioner recovers the woman's eggs, they are matured in a culture medium in an incubator. Some practitioners remove the outer membrane of the eggs to facilitate fertilisation. Semen is placed in the dish with the egg (or eggs) in another culture medium. This is a liquid mixture which provides the environment for egg survival and growth under laboratory conditions. It must mimic a woman's internal body as far as possible, so blood serum from the woman being treated might be used in the culture medium, and some reports state that a section of fallopian tube or uterine tissue was added. The culture medium contains antibiotics, which are not normally found in a woman's body, but necessary for *in vitro* survival of fertilised eggs. If fertilised, the single egg cell begins to divide slowly into two cells, four cells, and so on.

Embryo Transfer (ET) or Embryo Replacement (ER)

(Both terms are used by IVF practitioners. Many IVF teams use the term embryo transfer to mean any insertion of an *in vitro* embryo into a woman's womb. Edwards and Steptoe make a distinction. They use the term 'embryo replacement' when the woman who is receiving the embryo contributed her own egg, since to them 'embryo transfer' implies inserting the embryo into a woman who did not contribute her own egg. However, the term 'embryo replacement' is not accurate either. It sounds as if the embryo was already there in the woman's womb, removed, and then placed back. No IVF practitioners use the term 'embryo insertion', as I do.)

If fertilisation and cell growth proceed, and if the resulting embryo appears normal, at about the eight to twelve cell stage from one to five embryos are inserted into the woman's womb via a catheter (narrow tube) pushed through her cervix. The maximum number of embryos allowed to be inserted varies among IVF practitioners. The Voluntary Licensing Authority (VLA) in Britain recommends that no more than three fertilised eggs be inserted into the woman's womb at any one cycle. Ian Craft's IVF team at the private Wellington Hospital in London was inserting more than three, and quadruplets were born to one woman from his programme, the care of which was the responsibility of the National Health Service, not the private Wellington. Multiple births carry physical and emotional risks to mothers and babies. But Craft thought the VLA was going 'beyond its declared terms of reference' (Veitch, 1987c) in warning him to stop inserting more than three or four fertilised eggs into a woman, and threatening to take his licence away. Craft could still practise IVF without the approval of the VLA which has no legal authority. His team was also reducing the numbers of fetuses in the woman's womb by aborting some of them, which the VLA does not approve (Veitch, 1987a).

The embryo insertion procedure is considered simple and straightforward, but also a 'skill'. At least one IVF group, Richard Marrs' team in Los Angeles, has publicly reported their inability to insert embryos in some cases because of cervical blockage. Also, in all probability, this procedure contributes to the higher incidence of ectopic pregnancies in IVF.

At this stage, more hormones may be administered to the woman to aid implantation and pregnancy.

Few pregnancies result, and there is a high rate of miscarriage in IVF. The success rate of IVF is low. How low depends on who you talk to. In the early days of IVF, average 'liberal' estimates of overall 'success rates' were often given as 20–30 per cent. These figures quoted by practitioners made IVF sound effective as infertility treatment, but in fact they did not reflect that few women on IVF programmes have babies from this method. 'Success' is measured in a number of ways by IVF teams. Gena Corea and Susan Ince (1987) in the USA and Françoise Laborie (1987) in France have exposed the obvious manipulation of figures by IVF practitioners. Some clinics count as an IVF success the dubious 'chemical pregnancy', measured as a transient increase in the level of the hormone HCG in the woman's blood. This is not an established pregnancy at all; a woman does not even necessarily miss her period when a 'chemical pregnancy' has been proclaimed. Some clinics differentiate among laparoscopies to be used in statistics, depending on the effect it has on the statistics. Corea and Ince point out that in some USA clinics, if an initial laparoscopy ends in egg retrieval and a pregnancy, that laparoscopy is included in the reported figures. However, if an initial laparoscopy ends in no egg retrieval, then that laparoscopy is not represented in the statistics. Rather, it is portrayed as a preliminary step to accepting a woman on the IVF programme. In another example of 'massaging' the data, Corea and Ince found that some newly established IVF clinics in the USA have cited worldwide 'overall' success rates when advertising their own programmes where no pregnancies or births have been established. In 1985, the editor of the medical journal *Fertility and Sterility* berated his colleagues, writing that there 'is a failure of adherence to the highest ethical standard of truth in expressing the IVF pregnancy rate' (Soules, 1985, p. 511). In Britain, the second report of the Voluntary Licensing Authority, published in 1987, recorded tables of both IVF pregnancy rates and IVF live birth rates for the year 1985. Pregnancy was confirmed by ultrasound twenty-eight days after embryo insertion. The live birth percentage per treatment cycle for all IVF centres was 8.5 per cent. Now the admittedly quite low 'success rates' are being used by several IVF advocates to argue for more IVF experimentation, in order to increase the success rates.

If pregnancy does occur after embryo insertion, there is a greater chance with IVF of spontaneous abortion and ectopic pregnancy. If the woman does become pregnant, she is monitored by measuring hormone levels in blood and urine, and by pregnancy testing with blood tests and eventually ultrasound. Amniocentesis is routine for chromosome analysis of the gestating fetus. Most babies conceived by IVF are born by Caesarean section.

One woman may undergo many superovulations and laparosco-pies, since the success rate is low. IVF centres limit the number of laparoscopic egg retrievals per patient, for example, to five. The laparoscopy, though spoken of as routine, carries risks. The risks of the many manipulations are not discussed in any meaningful way by IVF practitioners or the media.

4

The domain of medicine

Infertility is a serious political problem. Many women with fertility problems demand the right to IVF treatment; many say they are happy to be a 'guinea pig' for medical science. IVF is not about infertility in particular, although IVF advocates have promoted it as such. In this chapter I explore more closely the application of IVF on women in the name of medical treatment, to show why it is not and never can be a *treatment* for fertility problems, and to show some of what IVF-as-medical-procedure is about.

I have kept in mind two arguments we often hear in favour of IVF. One, that IVF offers women a reproductive 'choice', and two, that IVF practitioners offer hope to women for whom no other hope exists. These are false claims, as we will see. It is inadequate to talk simply about 'choice'. Reproductive choices have repeatedly been taken away from women, women do not control what 'choices' are available, and the life decisions we do or do not make are effected by other social factors. Also, IVF does not address women's fertility problems as a *women's* health issue. There are women-respecting, positive approaches (other hopes) which can already be undertaken to address these problems.

Reproduction-the-domain-of-medicine

A 1986 definition of infertility from a World Health Organisation report illustrates a dominant medical view of women's reproduction, which confuses a normal pregnancy with an endangered one: 'A woman is considered infertile if she has been continuously

65

exposed to the *risk of pregnancy* for two years and has not conceived' (Diczfalusy, 1986, pp. 34–5, my emphasis). Reproductive technologies take that general outlook to its 'logical' end. The 'disfunctioning' body of women needs medical technology. There are women with fertility problems, women whose husbands have fertility problems, women who are able to reproduce but who have 'inferior' eggs, and so on and on. The number of medical conditions of reproduction expands with each new method of intervention. There is always something that can go 'wrong', as exemplified by the overuse of ultrasound scanning on pregnant women and Caesarean section on birthing women in many Western countries.[1] Barabara Katz Rothman commented, 'There's this incredible lack of faith in the body. We start feeling that we all need *in vitro* fertilisation and Caesarean sections to get babies in and out. And the natural reproductive process has been working just fine, thank you, for a real long time' (Hopkins, 1985).

IVF is a recent example in a long line of high-tech medical interventions applied to women's reproductive bodies. And the medical 'conditions' which are coming under its provenance are expanding.

Infertility is the first 'medical disability' for which IVF was put to use as a clinical treatment. As a clinical procedure, IVF was first used on women with damaged fallopian tubes.[2] From there, the medical indications for IVF multiplied rapidly. IVF is now being used in many countries:

— to treat women who are unable to reproduce from unknown causes, which accounts in some areas for almost one-third of women diagnosed as infertile;
— to treat women who are able to reproduce, but where there is a fertility problem in their male partners (sometimes called male subfertility, referring to poor sperm quality);
— to treat women with fertility problems due to endometriosis if the condition is relatively uncomplicated;
— to treat women without eggs, in conjunction with egg donation from another woman.

IVF, which was at first carefully sold to the public as a 'last resort' for women with blocked fallopian tubes, is now being considered for a myriad of other applications on women. In fact, by 1987 the percentage of women admitted to IVF programmes because of tubal problems is decreasing, while there is an increase worldwide in the number of women without fertility problems themselves who are being treated with IVF because of sperm problems in their partners (Laborie, 1988; National Perinatal Statistics Unit, 1987). Yet, few couples who enter IVF programmes are relieved from childlessness.

Genetic disease is the second 'medical disability' identified by IVF practitioners for treatment by IVF. Genetic applications of IVF include 'preimplantation screening', 'genetic therapy', 'egg donation', and 'sex pre-selection'. I will describe these genetic applications of IVF briefly here, and in greater detail in Chapter 6.

1. In June 1987, two laboratories in Britain announced that they had perfected methods for screening of IVF embryos for certain kinds of hereditary conditions and for sex (Veitch, 1987b; *The Guardian*, 1987b). The procedures, dubbed 'preimplantation screening', include:

— typing IVF embryos for chromosome normality and abnormality (chromosomes are structures in the cells where genes are packaged, which transmit hereditary information from one generation to the next; some disabilities occur with a specific chromosomal configuration, for example, Down's Syndrome);
— typing IVF embryos for sex (which may be predicted by looking at the 'sex chromosomes');
— analysing genes indirectly by looking at 'gene products', the chemicals produced by them (many pre-natal screening tests on the amniotic fluid extracted from a pregnant woman during amniocentesis use this method);
— analysing the genes directly with 'gene probes' for diagnostic screening of early embryos (each gene probe is a product of genetic engineering methods, and is specific for a certain condition or trait);

2. Genetic engineering methods are now used in animals for adding or altering genes in fertilised eggs; when this technique is used on women's eggs it is called 'gene therapy'. (As of September 1987 no laboratory has admitted to altering women's eggs using these methods, but it is a future prospect, as we will see in Chapters 6 and 8.)

3. Genetic application of IVF also includes using egg donation in women who are able to reproduce biologically, but who are 'carriers' of a genetic disease and so may give birth to a child with a condition, such as haemophilia;

4. Screening for the sex of an IVF embryo followed by selection of the desired sex is called sex determination. Another form of sex determination, more accurately called sex pre-determination, entails engineering the sex of the offspring at fertilisation. In 1986, a hospital in New Orleans (USA) announced that a male baby had been born using a combination of IVF and a sex pre-selection method.

Further, IVF methods have expanded the capabilities for genetic selection of embryos to include women who conceive in the usual way, that is, without egg removl and IVF. Using an embryo flushing method, the doctor tries to 'wash out' the fertilised egg before it implants in the women's uterine wall. With embryo in hand, the medical scientist can screen it with the battery of genetic screening tests, and then replace the embryo in the woman's womb if the embryo proves to be 'acceptable' by medical standards.

In short, IVF is being promoted for greater genetic control of reproduction. As one headline in the British daily, *The Guardian*, suggested, 'Couples will be able to check "healthy" embryos' (Veitch, 1987b). Actually, it is the medical scientist who will decide which embryos are 'healthy', and of course what constitutes 'healthy'. IVF is not merely a procedure aimed at fertility management, as they say. IVF is also a 'check' on many women's reproduction. And as I will show below, the number of conditions considered genetic in origin is growing, and the number of conditions considered 'preventable' by screening is also growing. This means that more and more women are targeted as 'needing' IVF and embryo flushing to reproduce.

The scope of *in vitro* reproduction is unlimited. The uses of IVF for medical management of infertility in couples and for genetic 'disease' have opened the door to the inclusion of every other scientific discipline of reproduction known to the realm of IVF practice and research. These include research into embryo nutrition, immunological aspects of egg fertilisation and embryo development, the quest for new contraceptives, and more. Infertility-the-medical-condition is not the target of IVF. Women's reproduction is.

Infertility-the-excuse

The use on women of superovulation, egg removal, fertilisation of eggs in laboratories, insertion of fertilised eggs in women's wombs, and subsequent failures or success at creating babies by IVF could not proceed without naming medical conditions in need of treatment, for obvious ethical reasons. Infertility provided medical scientists with the first such medical condition.

Government inquiries on IVF issues accept this. The British Warnock Report introduced IVF issues with this assessment:

> an inability to have children is a malfunction . . . In addition, the psychological distress that may be caused by infertility in those who want children may precipitate a mental disorder warranting treatment. It is, in our view, *better to treat the primary cause* of such distress than to alleviate the symptoms. (Warnock Report, 1984, p. 9, my emphasis)

Notice that by the 'primary cause' they did not mean the causes of infertility. They consider infertility in itself to be the *primary* cause of people's distress. By taking this approach, they could bypass a discussion of the known causes of infertility and prevention, and of the broader social questions of the distress of infertility, what motherhood is about, why many women and men feel a great need to be biological parents, and so on. They accepted a specialist, high-tech medical/scientific approach for fixing infertility-the-cause.

The popular media support this meaning generally, quoting doctors and the IVF 'experts' themselves. Dr Robert Winston, a British infertility specialist and IVF practitioner at Hammersmith Hospital in London wrote in *The Observer* newspaper: 'Infertility is actually a terrible disease, affecting our sexuality and well-being. Marriages disintegrate and even suicide is not unknown' (Winston, 1985). He wrote this, not to suggest complex psychosocial reasons for the problems; not to call for better public health measures against the growing environmental and iatrogenic (doctor-induced) causes of infertility; not to call for more adequate primary health care for treatment of infections which are a major cause of infertility in women. He wrote this article to argue for what he and every other IVF advocate calls 'human embryo research', that is, experimentation using women's bodies. A long article on artificial reproduction in the US news weekly *Time*, in 1984, similarly identified infertility as a marriage wrecker and saw a need for highly skilled 'experts' in artificial reproduction technology to combat the present infertility epidemic.

Some couples' relationships do suffer because of their fertility problems. However, others also express that their fertility problems bring them closer together. And many women are speaking out about their deep emotional and psychological experiences of infertility. But citing these problems the way IVF advocates do, to support the use of IVF on women, is not an appreciation of the social and cultural dimensions of infertility, or the prices which IVF entails. It is a platitude, an excuse.

IVF is offered as the final hope for couples who cannot reproduce. What was never made clear enough from the beginning, however, is that every kind of fertility problem does not come under the IVF umbrella. Complicated fertility problems are not considered by medical 'experts' as treatable by IVF, for example, for women with blocked tubes plus endometriosis or endocrine problems, or for women with chlamydia trachomatis infections. (*Chlamydia* is a micro-organism which is a cause of pelvic inflammatory disease, an infection of the upper reproductive tract. Its incidence among women in Western countries is increasing at an alarming rate.) Another fact which is not made clear enough is that many women on IVF clinic waiting lists have become pregnant without ever starting the programme. In other words, whatever their fertility problem was, it was not necessary to undergo IVF to reproduce.

IVF does not cure infertility. IVF does not heal women's blocked tubes or the subfertility in men. It does nothing to answer the question of infertility from 'unknown causes'. In fact, IVF carries a risk of causing fertility problems in women, many of whom have no fertility problem in the first place. IVF is highly invasive biochemically and surgically; the powerful drugs and manipulation of internal organs are known causes of reproductive system damage.

IVF is a 'technical fix' in that it bypasses the *causes* of fertility problems. IVF is not going to change the fertility problems of women, if anything it is going to make them worse. Most importantly, this is not the way it has to be. Many of the causes of infertility are known *and preventable*. Some of the most obvious preventable causes come from cervical cancer, from reproductive tract infections which have not been diagnosed and treated properly, from doctor-prescribed contraceptives and sloppy abdominal surgery, and from lack of information given to women on known and probable causes. Despite this knowledge, the British Government's Warnock Inquiry started from the understanding that infertility-is-the-cause of a medical problem and IVF is an acceptable way to fix it. They did not recognise the known, preventable causes of infertility as of medical interest.

Some of the known preventable causes of infertility are:[3]

Infection

Infections from pelvic inflammatory disease (PID) and sexually transmitted disease cause scarring of the fallopian tubes when not treated soon enough. PIDs are infections of the uterus, fallopian tubes and ovaries; they are considered major causes of both ectopic pregnancy and infertility due to tubal damage. A World Health Organisation study showed that among women diagnosed as infertile, 50.9 per cent of those with a previous history of PID had an infection-related diagnosis (Diczfalusy, 1986, p. 38). Why are all those governments and doctors who are so concerned about infertility not calling for a concerted screening effort for women most at risk? The World Health Organisation 1978 Task Force on the Diagnosis and Treatment of Infertility identified infections as *preventable* causes of fertility problems globally.

For example, the contraceptive intrauterine device (IUD) is a direct cause of infertility. Many women are at risk; a United Nations global survey from the mid-1980s showed that 12 per cent of women used IUDs (Anderson, 1985). A direct correlation between IUDs and infertility was known in the mid-1970s. In 1978, the *British Medical Journal* reported that IUD users have a threefold increase in fallopian tube inflammation; a higher proportion of miscarriage and ectopic pregnancies if they do become pregnant; and a high risk of infertility in women who have never given birth (the same correlation was not found in women who had given birth before using the IUD). Two different 1985 studies from the USA proved the causal link between the IUD and infertility beyond a doubt. Both studies showed that using the IUD doubles the risk of becoming infertile because of a resulting PID.

Other infections which are significant causes of infertility in women today are the PID *Chlamydia trachomatis*, prevalent in Western countries, and genital tuberculosis which is prevalent in Africa and Asia.

At least since the late 1970s, some doctors have recognised the need for wider diagnostic facilities for genital infections that could become PIDs. Medical studies have also shown that abortion increases the risk of later fertility problems in women who have undiagnosed genital infections. Again, preliminary diagnosis and treatment of these infections would be a sound preventive measure. Post-abortion infection is another cause of infertility. The need for high standards and adequate facilities for abortion services is obvious.

Hormonal drugs of contraception and pregnancy intervention

Hormonal drugs, including oral contraceptives, long-lasting inject- able contraceptives, and 'morning after' pills are also known causes of reproductive tract abnormalities and pregnancy complications.

For one, DES (diethylstilbestrol, a synthetic estrogen) was frequently given to pregnant women in the 1950s and 1960s as a miscarriage prevention drug. It was never proven effective in preventing miscarriages (Direcks, 1987). The daughters of women who were prescribed the drug during pregnancy are now having associated fertility problems, a high rate of miscarriage and ectopic pregnancies, tubal abnormalities and cancer. It is still used today as a 'morning after pill'.

Another example is Depo Provera, a synthetic progesterone. As a long-lasting injectable contraceptive, it is designed to be administered to women once every three months. It has never been approved as a contraceptive in the USA; but it is licensed for long-term use in Britain as a 'last resort' contraceptive. Depo Provera has also been widely promoted by international aid agencies for use on women in Bangladesh and other 'Third World' countries as part of population control strategies. Little is known of its long-term effects, but they may include alterations to a woman's immunological system and congenital problems if the drug remains in a woman's system while she is pregnant. Immediate possible effects include cessation of menstrual bleeding or excessive or irregular bleeding, weight gain or loss, headaches, dizziness, depression, back pain, stomach discomfort, nausea, breast tenderness, tiredness, and difficulty in getting pregnant for eight months to two years after the last injection.

In spite of medical evidence, in a 1984 US medical school textbook, *Current Therapy in Infertility*, Dr George Huggins wrote that the reproductive implications of the IUD and the contraceptive Pill are not so bad, and that problems associated with abortion arise because women do not listen to their doctors. The book was edited by top names in obstetrics and gynaecology, including Luigi Mastroianni, the director of the IVF programme at the Hospital of the University of Pennsylvania (Garcia *et al.*, 1984).

Cervical cancer

Cervical cancer, becoming more widespread in young women, can lead to loss of the cervix and possibly the uterus if not treated in time. Diagnosis of cervical cancer, and cervical abnormalities which precede cancer, is relatively straightforward. In Britain, some doctors and epidemiologists, health care workers, women's support groups and reproductive rights activists are calling for an organised screening policy for PIDs and cervical cancer, and demanding that women be given all available medical information about the known causes of cervical cancer, so that we may make informed decisions about our life-styles. For example, two factors which increase a woman's chance of cervical cancer are smoking and taking the contraceptive Pill. According to Jean Robinson, a lay member of the General Medical Council who has thoroughly researched the epidemiological history of cervical cancer in Britain, the correlation between the Pill and cervical cancer has been purposely suppressed by the medical profession (Robinson, 1987). Doctors who objected to giving women the information told Robinson that they were afraid women might stop taking oral contraceptives.

The problem in the above cases is not lack of knowledge and ability, but commitment and lack of political will among the policy-makers, funding bodies, and doctors who wish to control women's behaviour by suppressing information.

The lack of response to these known causes of infertility by policy-makers and government inquiries into IVF is telling.

Environmental toxins

Environmental and workplace pollution are other known causes of fertility problems in women and men. A large number of industrially produced toxins and radiations are known to present reproductive hazards, and there is growing evidence that visual display units (VDUs, also called visual display terminals) are also associated with women's fertility problems (Huws, 1987). There is, in addition, the increased chance of associated congenital problems in offspring due to hazards in the workplace. Not all congenital or 'at birth' conditions are inherited; much is due to a random gene mutation (a chance occurrence during one particular pregnancy), environmental factors, illness, and medical treatment. Industrial pollution and waste is one source, as in the Love Canal case in the USA. The Love Canal residents lived in the vicinity of a toxic waste dump and many suffered chromosomal damage and congenital health problems from the chemicals leaking out of the dump.

Another source of reproductive hazards is the presence of ionising radiation in the environment from atomic energy installations and wastage dumps (as in the area near Buffalo, New York, where many women are infertile due to heavy radioactive fallout) and radioactive contamination from nuclear weapons testing (such as the US atomic bomb experiments in the South Pacific around the Marshall Islands in the 1950s).

The above examples and others have been well documented (see Bertell, 1985; Denning, 1985; Elkington, 1986; Hynes, 1987; Kee, 1987; Huws, 1987).

It should be clear by now that if doctors and reproductive biologists and governments are so concerned with helping women and men with fertility problems and with preventing congenital conditions in offspring, there are sensible and effective measures that may be taken to prevent them. The medical profession could be treating a medical condition such as PID. Or epidemiologists could be identifying reproductive hazards in the workplace and environment – which could be changed, but at a cost. This is not to say that such an alternative approach would be sufficient to address all fertility problems, or the emotional dimensions of fertility and motherhood, or that these measures would by themselves bring about women's reproductive autonomy and sexual freedom. But they are necessary steps.

Of course, to do all this would mean a change in the medical–science approach. Taking the women's health route, instead of the technical fix route, would help women as a group most. But this is not a Nobel Prize winning project. It would not feed into the burgeoning biotechnology industry. It would give women more control over our own reproduction, and not less, the way doctor-controlled reproduction does. And these are major reasons why we are given the IVF/genetic engineering 'choices', but not other choices.

Some fertility problems are not as obviously preventable as those mentioned above. Acute endometriosis and hormonal imbalance accounts for a significant amount of infertility, and a small percentage of women are missing reproductive organs from birth. Known preventive measures may not address some of these problems, but for most of these cases neither will IVF. For women whose tubes are damaged today because of infection, all the prevention in the world will not help now. It is true that for some of these women, IVF is a last hope for becoming pregnant and giving birth. And some women, though not many, do finally achieve that end. According to the Voluntary Licensing Authority in Britain, in 1985, 364 women gave birth to babies out of 3717 women undergoing IVF treatment, in a total of 4308 attempts called 'treatment cycles'.[4] The question is, how can we be willing to accept all that high-tech reproduction means for that? IVF cannot be understood in a vacuum. The time, effort, expense, and most importantly the medical point of view which high-tech (scientific) reproduction entails means that to proceed with IVF research and clinical practice, thousands and thousands of women must undergo this kind of reproduction. IVF is not particularly about infertility, as should be clear from the above discussion. IVF, growing eggs and embryos outside the female body and in laboratories, is first a technology of so-called 'pure' research aimed at a specific kind of knowledge acquisition and also aimed at technological control of all sorts of reproductive processes. It is about reproductive engineering of the most extreme kind, as the US Government recognised early on in the IVF debate (see quote, p. 16).

Who is 'fit' to breed

Reproduction is historically the most potent area of social control of women. Control of women's sexuality and reproduction is tied up in cultural notions of marriage and kinship, family, 'blood' relationship – the very foundations of social organisation. The rise of obstetrics and gynaecology as a male medical profession in Europe and North America brought women's reproductive lives into the medical domain. Making *all* pregnancy and childbirth a medical condition, not only endangered pregnancies, brought with it the role of medical professionals as social, moral and technical authorities over reproduction, and so over women. The authority of doctors and now medical scientists is not monolithic, but it is powerful as exemplified by the growing medical authority over women in the name of 'fetal health' (see Chapter 2). For other examples, in Britain women must receive permission from two doctors to have an abortion; medical authorities define the criteria for eugenic abortion (which women should be allowed to undergo amniocentesis for pre-natal screening), and whether or not single women should be eligible for artificial insemination programmes (see Steinberg, 1987).

The new artificial reproduction technologies extend that medical authority further. These social control aspects of the new reproductive and genetic technologies ride on the wave of IVF-the-infertility-treatment.

Medical articles and reports on IVF practice on women, whether from Britain, Australia, or the USA carefully mention that the practitioners are treating married or 'stable' cohabiting heterosexual couples. The term 'wife' is often used when talking about the woman undergoing treatment even when the couple is not married. The label 'wife' is not used in medical reports for treatment of other medical conditions, of course.

Further, the medical profession has stressed its authority to choose which infertile couples are eligible for IVF treatment. The British Medical Association (BMA) IVF guidelines state that treatment should only be undertaken after assessment of the stability of the familial relationship of the couple. In an article on medicine and the law for the medical journal *The Lancet*, barrister Diana Brahams concurred with this extension of doctors' social authority in matters of IVF reproduction. She wrote: 'When a woman presents [herself] for treatment with IVF, the doctor should keep in mind the interests of the child he [sic] is helping to create. Thus either marriage or stable relationship is desirable, and particularly, where there is donated ova or sperm, the character of the potential parents should be kept in mind.' Brahams noted that the 'natural process' of reproducing takes no regard for this level of doctor-control, but that with IVF 'there is the possibility of control' (Brahams, 1983, p. 729).

Similarly, the Royal College of Obstetricians and Gynaecologists (RCOG) stated in their 1983 guidelines on IVF that doctors have the right to refuse treatment on social as well as medical grounds. The Report of the Ethics Committee on *In Vitro* Fertilisation and Embryo Replacement (ER) or Transfer stated that 'it would be wrong arbitrarily to exclude all single women from IVF and ER without consideration of their individual circumstances' (RCOG, 1983, p. 7). But this thought from the RCOG is merely a cautious point. It protects them from any suggestion of discrimination against single women, but it does not constrain their authority to choose who is fit to breed. The report summary states that IVF should 'be used for single women only in exceptional circumstances' (p. 18), never naming the circumstances. (Perhaps a single woman doctor or lawyer would be deemed socially 'fit'?) While discussing eligibility outside marriage, they assert, 'most practitioners will intuitively feel that IVFand ER should be performed in the most "natural" of family environments', that is marriage (p. 6).

The RCOG report extends the authority of doctors to make social and moral decisions about which women are socially fit to breed in the context of IVF. They stress that the doctor is the final authority. Most explicitly they emphasize that IVF doctors are not only 'enablers', but are also taking part in the formation of the embryo itself, and so will have a 'special sense of responsibility for the welfare of the child thus conceived' (p. 6).

Greater control of women's reproduction means greater quality control of embryos, too. A hand-out sheet distributed by the pro-life (anti-abortion) group at the University of York made the inaccurate, woman-blaming charge, 'Already test-tube mothers can dispose of and reject potentially handicapped embryos.' Women do not have control over IVF embryos. IVF practitioners do. In the informed consent agreement recommended for use by the Voluntary Licensing Authority in Britain, the *couple* in a licensed

IVF programme sign an agreement which stipulates 'selection by the medical and scientific staff of the most suitable pre-embryos [sic] for such replacement [into the woman's womb]' (MRC/RCOG VLA Report, 1986, p. 41).

Practitioners often stress the social usefulness of IVF: IVF saves marriages; IVF makes families 'complete'; IVF makes 'better' babies (that is, genetically related and genetically screened); even that IVF couples make better parents. In the medical journal *Fertility and Sterility*, Ian Johnston's IVF team at the University of Melbourne and The Royal Women's Hospital, Carlton in Australia wrote: 'There is more love and tolerance exhibited in these marriages [infertile marriages] than in the vast majority of fertile marriages, and *in vitro* fertilisation offers many of these couples their one opportunity for complete fulfillment (Johnston *et al.*, 1981, p. 704). Patrick Steptoe similarly wrote that the birth of Louise Brown to Lesley and John Brown made 'this family complete at long last' (Steptoe, 1980b, p. 181), despite the fact that Lesley and John Brown were the parents of a child from John's previous marriage.

IVF promotes the 'superiority' of a genetic relationship. When a 'true' genetic relationship is not possible, IVF can provide a second best alternative by matching 'genetic traits' of egg and sperm donors. IVF can make nuclear families complete, even to the point of promising a certain race and complexion. In the *British Medical Journal*, Alan Trounson and his IVF team at Monash University and Queen Victoria Medical Centre in Melbourne wrote, 'A frozen sample of semen, matched to the recipient's husband's physical characteristics (race, complexion, build, height, eye colour, and blood group) was thawed' (Trounson *et al.*, 1983, p. 836).

The 'socially useful' procedure of 'matching' traits reflects racial and patriarchal attitudes about paternity and the importance of making the child appear to be have a 'blood relationship'. In 1984, just three months after the Warnock Report was published in Britain, Wood and Trounson's IVF team discussed how IVF is better than old-fashioned adoption in an article in the *British Medical Journal* entitled 'Clinical Developments in *In Vitro* Fertilisation':

> Prenatal adoption of unwanted embryos may have advantages over postnatal adoption. Matching of donors and recipients may be more accurate, as adoption agencies are restricted . . . The

recipient of the embryo experiences the emotional changes of pregnancy and birth, and the mother–child relationship may be favourably influenced by these and the early postnatal experiences. (Wood *et al.*, 1984, p. 980)

Their assessment is biologistic and insulting to adopting parents. Certainly pregnancy and childbirth is a profound and sensuous experience, with great meaning. But this kind of measuring and fixing and codifying of concepts has nothing to do with the appreciation of women's experiences. Just the opposite. Their attitude removes the experience as women's and takes it out-of-women's-control. They define the parent–child relationship in one dimension, making a biological–genetic experience so meaningful that it necessitates invasion and control of women's reproduction by 'experts'. Here, the biological is reduced to a *particular* experience, ignoring other kinds of sensuous, physical (i.e. biological) relationships.

Medical and science 'experts' are moulding cultural norms to their so-called 'objective' knowledge. They have a power to define the problems, the therapies, the technology, and its social meaning. Most obviously, the word 'mother' is often used to identify the woman on an IVF programme, both in the medical/science literature and in oral discussion. This struck me at a talk by Dr Henry Leese, a researcher who collaborates with Robert Edwards on a human embryo research project. In a lecture on the clinical procedures involved in IVF, delivered to science teachers at the 1986 Annual Meeting of the Association for Science and Education at the Uiversity of York, he said the *mother is superovulated*. Do our menstrual rhythms make us all mothers? This usage was perhaps picked up from Robert Edwards; in a 1970 article Edwards co-authored with Steptoe and Jean Purdy, they wrote: 'Human oocytes [eggs] have been taken from the mother before ovulation' (Edwards, Steptoe and Purdy, 1970, p. 1307). It would be eight more years before any woman whose eggs they took would become a mother by the method. Such misrepresentation by many IVF practitioners is not helpful to women underoing the procedures. By equating women's physiology and biochemistry to motherhood, the language fits an idea that biology is destiny. It is subtle and powerful. It subverts women's own motherhood. In *Of Women Born*, the feminist poet Adrienne Rich wrote:

What makes us mothers? The care of small children? The physical changes of pregnancy and birth? What of the woman who, never having been pregnant, begins lactating when she adopts an infant? What of the women who . . . has practically raised her younger sisters and brothers?[5]

The message coming from advocates of IVF and related procedures such as egg donation is that they are socially useful because they can 'fix' women's biology to fit into narrow, patriarchal images of women's social role. Many couples on IVF programmes are not childless people. Many have had children from previous relationships, but cannot reproduce as a couple. Despite everything that IVF entails for women, it is acceptable to include couples who already have children partly because making 'better babies' (genetically related or genetically matched) for couples solidifies the class interests of the medical profession as a whole, and it stabilises patriarchal social relations. Any woman unattached to a man, lesbians and single women, are virtually ineligible for IVF, for this is not 'socially useful'. (In addition, a former prostitute was refused IVF treatment at St. Mary's Hospital in Manchester because she was considered unsuitable to become a mother (Boseley, 1987)). No IVF 'expert' is arguing that the new reproductive technologies will allow women reproductive autonomy.

Clearly, IVF and the new reproductive technolgies allow doctors more control, women less control, over reproduction. Sheila Kitzinger, who writes and lectures on birth and motherhood, reported a case in Britain where women protested against a male obstetrician from the 'doctor knows best' school:

In 1982 the Professor of Obstetrics[6] at the Royal Free Hospital announced that in future all women in his unit must deliver lying down. There was a spontaneous uprising among women and 5,000 people gathered on Parliament Hill fields in protest. Shortly after, the professor resigned and went into *in vitro* fertilisation. His leaving, he said, was nothing to do with the protests. (Kitzinger, 1985)

Well, women are easier to control in IVF, and embryos do not talk back.

Choice according to IVF

IVF advocates eventually mention women as active participants in IVF in the context of 'choice'. IVF practitioners, from Steptoe and Edwards in England to Carl Wood and Alan Trounson's group in Australia, repeatedly uphold the right of women to 'choose' IVF. The complexities of the issue of choice are not dealt with by these same men. Their spoken concerns for women's right to chose exist only within IVF.

They use pro-woman sounding statements selectively. When criticised by Edwards and Steptoe for allowing a 42-year-old woman into an IVF programme, Wood and Trounson defended the right of over-40-year-old women to make an informed decision about IVF (Trounson *et al.*, 1983b). Yet, Carl Wood and colleagues appeased right-to-lifers with the statement, 'the whole point of freezing embryos is to preserve life, not destroy it' (Walters and Singer, 1982, p. 38). Similarly, the Italian IVF practitioner Domenico Geraci said, 'If the Church opposes abortion, it should be in sympathy with our work' (*New Scientist*, 1982b, p. 7). Playing into the rhetoric of anti-abortionists is hardly sensitive to women's right to choose.

We similarly hear the argument that women should have the 'free' choice to become 'surrogates' if we want to. But what does that mean? One survey showed that 40 per cent of women who became 'surrogate' mothers were unemployed or on welfare (Winslade, 1981). In the USA, where the commercial surrogacy industry flourishes, it is obvious that payment matters. Gena Corea interviewed John Stehura, president of the Bionetics Foundation Inc., an organisation in the surrogate mother business. He admitted that when surrogacy becomes a more common practice, the surrogate industry can then hire poor women who will accept lower fees. He added that when 'embryo flushing' becomes common, poor women from Mexico and Central America could be procured as 'surrogate' mothers, his point being that the woman will not be donating any of her genetic material (eggs). The racist underpinnings of the embryo flushing/surrogate mother method is that a woman from Mexico or Central America is fine for gestating an embryo created with an egg from a White, North American woman (Corea, 1985; Arditti, 1987).

Folklore and anthropologists tell us that women have carried children for other women in the past, though more often in other societies and cultures. This is not the same as the phenomenon of 'surrogacy' which is happening as an offshoot to the new reproductive technologies. 'Surrogate motherhood' as the relatively recent phenomenon in industrialised countries emerged along with the new reproductive technologies. As 'surrogacy' is meant today, it is an adaptation on women of methods used on laboratory and agricultural animals, for example in the dairy and meat industries to create greater numbers of a selected strain of cows. (A female animal may be artificially inseminated with sperm from a prized male, or else she might be impregnated with IVF embryos created from 'superior strains' of cows.) Taking the technique to the realm of medicine, a woman may be inseminated with sperm from a male contractor, or else an IVF embryo created from the egg of a woman who cannot conceive and the sperm of her partner might be inserted into a 'carrying mother's' womb. The medicalisation of surrogacy is not equivalent to the non-technological examples coming from other cultures.

The majority of the British Warnock Committee favoured banning surrogacy, and the 1985 Surrogacy Arrangements Act criminalised commercial surrogacy in Britain. However, many British doctors and IVF practitioners oppose such a blanket rejection of surrogacy. They would accept it as a womb-for-therapy. In 1985, a small majority of British doctors voted in favour of surrogacy-for-therapy at the annual meeting of the British Medical Association, against the BMA's official policy. In 1986, Edwards and Steptoe announced their opinion that surrogacy should be allowed for certain cases within their IVF programme. The journal *Nature* attacked the ban on surrogacy in an editorial, suggesting a solution to the whole problem. They proposed that corporations with the legal status of charities should control surrogacy (*Nature*, 1986). This is another example of how scientists presume to speak in the organisation of society. 'Surrogacy', the use of women as breeders, has been reinvented by doctors and scientists as an allied medical practice.

With the medicalisation of surrogacy, doctors reserve the right to judge a reproductive 'option'. Calling surrogacy a 'therapy' for infertility masks the nature of surrogacy arrangements. The 'surrogate mother' is providing a child of her labour, not a medical therapy for infertility.

The concepts 'reproductive rights' and 'reproductive choice' have been co-opted by medical science and other agents of the state to advocate medical/scientist controlled, technological reproduction. No one has a 'right' to children by *any* means; doctors should have no 'right' to make eugenic decisions about who is 'fit' to breed.

In a talk 'How the New Reproductive Technologies Frame Choices for Women' at the conference Women, Reproduction and Technology in Oxford, in 1987, Christine Crowe placed the feminist concept of 'choice' in its context. She reminded us that one of the main tenets of the women's movement has been the issue of choice in relation to sexuality and reproduction, 'The concept of the right to choose arose as a short-hand way for putting forward for women in industrialised countries the desire for the option to determine our own reproductive capacity.' For women in industrialised countries 'choice' revolved around the question of abortion. But for women in 'Third World' countries, and for Black, disabled and poor women in industrialised countries, 'choice' was not the issue, but rather how to resist sterilisation abuse, eugenic abortion, and the lack of options in contraceptive practice.

The most important questions for women are, why are we given *some* 'choices' and not others, and why are certain women allowed to decide among a particular set of reproductive options, while other women are not. For women now and in future faced with these new reproductive and genetic technologies, including genetic engineering technologies, the question of choice goes deeper than 'IVF on demand', or 'genetic engineering on demand'. Health care is not equivalent to technological capability.

Robyn Rowland suggests that for feminists, the 'right to choose' is better understood as our demand for the 'right to control' our own bodies. 'We have then to ask whether the new reproductive technologies give women greater control over our lives' (Rowland, 1987, p. 72).

5

The status of scientific knowledge

IVF pioneer Robert Edwards relates that he became interested in the possibility of *in vitro* fertilisation in mammals in the late 1950s, 'aroused by work on the superovulation of mice' and 'the explosion of knowledge of human chromosomes' (Edwards, 1983a, p. 55). He was inspired by the potential of using invasive drug regimens and the up and coming science of genetics. He voiced no early interest in women's health issues.

In this chapter I look at the use of women as experimental material for laboratory research into reproduction, in particular by IVF doctors and scientists for the pursuit of scientific knowledge. I wish to show how reproductive researchers use women's bodies as the 'raw materials' of scientific inquiry, although these same doctors and scientists, and their apologists, accept these activities as ethical, progressive, and necessary. As we will see, the pursuit of scientific knowledge on women's bodies follows 'logically' within the scientific approach to reproduction, which is to say it is not a 'monster' phenomenon but part of a whole culture of science in need of radical change.

The use of women as experimental material in IVF research does not 'simply' follow from the biological fact that women bear children. Biological facts do not speak for themselves; they exist within a social context, amidst cultural beliefs and norms. There are two points to make here. First, historically, women have been the subject of social intervention in reproduction. Invasive techniques of modern contraception, such as hormonal contraceptives and the IUD, are directed at women in Western, industrialised countries, and at women in 'Third World' countries, who are the major targets of population control strategies. This is, of course, historically consistent with the social control of women's sexual behaviour in order to control our reproductive activity: who has children, and under what circumstances. The use of women for IVF fits in with the common idea in patriarchy that women are the targets of reproductive control.

Second, the scientific approach to 'human reproduction' is not a unique discipline. It fits within the study of reproduction in other mammals. The use of women's bodies as experimental material is an extension of the similar use of female animals in reproductive science. Neither is this a simple biological 'fact' of nature (females reproduce the species). On the contrary, the similar use of animals and women in reproductive research stems from the relationship of the scientist (as intellectual Man) and the object of study, nature. In the pursuit of 'human reproduction', woman is that object of study. The relationship of scientist-subject to nature-object is a legacy of the Enlightenment visionaries, Descartes and Bacon.[1] And as the historian Carolyn Merchant discovered in her study of original writings of these men, the image of woman-as-nature verus man-as-observer was firmly entrenched in their world view (Merchant, 1982).

Today, this confrontational relationship between Man [sic] and living nature is magnified as a result of social conditions, of the capitalist-patriarchy that fuels the invention of marketable technologies for reproductive engineering. Certainly, the last two centuries have seen an increasing exploitation of the environment within capitalist culture. On the use of animals in industralised countries, John Berger (1980, p. 14) writes, 'Animals are always the observed. The fact that they can observe us has lost all significance. They are the objects of our ever-extending knowledge. What we know about them is an index of our power, and thus an index of what separates us from them.'

The new reproductive technologies have expanded what can be done to animals. Now, embryo transfer, *in vitro* fertilisation, gamete intrafallopian transfer (GIFT) and their permutations are being used in animal husbandry on cows, sheep, pigs, horses and in laboratory research on rabbits, hamsters, mice, rats, guinea pigs, and more (see Corea, 1985; Vines, 1987).

Because the scientific approach to reproduction likens women's reproduction to that of animals, it ignores, does not even see, the relevence of women's humanity, that is, women's diverse and active experiences of female fertility, pregnancy and childbirth. How is this possible? In *Patriarchy and Accumulation on a World Scale* Maria Mies (1986, p. 23) explains:

> By the dualistic splitting up of sex and gender, however, by treating the one [sex] as biological and the other [gender] as cultural, the door is again opened for those who want to treat the sexual difference between humans as a matter of our anatomy or as 'matter'. Sex as matter can then become an object for the scientist who may dissect, analyse, manipulate and reconstruct it according to his plans . . . This sphere can become a new hunting ground for biological engineering, for reproduction-technology, for genetic and eugenic engineering and last but not least for capital accumulation.

In the scientific approach to reproduction, women lose status as human subject. According to the scientist, biologically we are like sheep and cows. Thus, the reproductive engineer enjoys status as THE human subject. In IVF the acting, creative subject is the IVF doctor or scientist, revealingly referred to as the 'test-tube' father.

Women as experimental subject, not human subject

The following look at some of the early attempts to grow eggs and fertilised eggs in laboratories is not an attempt at a complete history of IVF and embryo transfer, nor is it definitive. But whether the first 'successful' fertilisation of a woman's egg in a laboratory occurred in 1948 by Menkin and Rock (as some IVF 'experts' maintain) or 1966 by Edwards and colleagues (as others maintain) does not matter for my purpose here, which is to expose the use of women as experimental subjects in IVF research.[2]

Embryo transfer preceded IVF in the reproductive scientist's repertoire of established *in vitro* methods. In 1890, Walter Heape, a British scientist working in Cambridge, transferred embryos removed from a pregnant Angora rabbit doe to the uterus of a Belgian hare doe. The hare gave birth to Angora rabbits and the first successful embryo transfer was reported. Between 1929 and 1933, scientific papers reported attempts to maintain embryos *in vitro* acquired from inside the bodies of female rabbits, guinea pigs and rats. By 1959, British scientists Anne McLaren and John Biggers reported their success with embryo culture (growing embryos in the laboratory under artificial conditions) and embryo transfer using mice. These types of experiments required embryos – that is, eggs which were fertilised in the female body; these embryos were removed from the pregnant female animal who is usually killed during the operation.

The first published report of IVF appeared in 1880 by the Viennese embryologist S. L. Schenk. He used eggs taken from the ovaries of rabbits and guinea pigs. Some years later another scientist reported IVF attempts on eggs of rabbits and guinea pigs; his report was published some time after the experiments, in 1893. Both these nineteenth-century men of science reported successes at fertilisation *in vitro*. Their 'successes' were later disregarded by scientists since there was no concrete proof that fertilisation had taken place.

Known attempts to culture eggs extracted from women's bodies date from 19335 with the published report of Gregory Pincus and B. V. Enzmann in the USA. Much of the early work on mammalian IVF in the USA was associated with them and Harvard University. No credible fertilisation of animal (mammal) eggs preceded Pincus and Enzmann's experiments using women's eggs, although in 1934 they published what they believed was the 'first certain demonstration that mammalian eggs can be fertilised *in vitro*' (quoted in Menkin and Rock's discussion, 1948, p. 440). In 1948, Miriam Menkin and John Rock, from Harvard Medical School and the Fertility Clinic Laboratories of the Free Hospital for Women, reported successful *in vitro* fertilisation of women's eggs. In 1955, Landrum Shettles, from the Department of Obstetrics and Gynaecology at Columbia University and the Sloan Hospital for Women in New York, published his own 'success' with IVF using women's eggs. These reported 'successes' at fertilisation *in vitro* were later disregarded (see Edwards discussion, 1983a, p. 56).

Work proceeded in the USA and Britain on egg and sperm interaction using animals. In 1959, Min-Cheuh Chang, also working in the USA alongside Gregory Pincus, reported what is today considered by many the first successful fertilisation *in vitro*, on rabbit egg and sperm. In 1964, Chang and Yanagimachi reported success using IVF with hamster egg and sperm. According to Robert Edwards (Ibid., p. 59), Yanagimachi and Chang's work with hamsters, the only applicable IVF 'successs' to speak of, guided his work at Cambridge using women's eggs. In other words, work on eggs taken from women proceeded although scientists had no understanding of the processes of mammalian egg maturation and fertilisation. Edwards proceeded with his work on women's eggs based on the singular success in hamsters. Reviewing the history of IVF attempts using mammalian eggs, Edwards said of Menkin, Rock and Shettles, those IVF pioneers who preceded him:

> But their work was not established on any fundamental knowledge of oocyte [egg] maturation, fertilisation *in vitro* and the culture of mammalian embryos *in vitro*. Without such understanding, progress was doomed to be very limited and no authentic examples of fertilisation can be accepted . . . There was little point, for example, in collecting oocytes from the oviduct [fallopian tube], because there would be no prior knowledge on the time of ovulation and the oocytes rapidly become degenerate. (Ibid., p. 56)

Pincus, Rock and Chang eventually diverted from their IVF studies, turning their collective attention to finding a hormonal contraceptive which would inhibit ovulation. This became known as the Pill. As a consultant for the pharmaceutical company Searle, the scientist Pincus and his medical associate gynaecologist John Rock collaborated on the first large-scale clinical trials of the Pill on Puerto Rican and Haitian women. Those trials were later brought into disrepute for their racist use of women in developing countries, and for damaging health as a result of the experiments, including cases of associated deaths in women (Seaman and Seaman, 1978). Feminists were instrumental in bringing these criticisms to light, and for making it clear that underlying such approaches to birth control is the presumption that women's sexuality and reproduction must be controlled to suit men's sexuality, where women are the locus of population control strategies. I mention this to show the links among reproductive technologies. The scientific approach to reproductive physiology points to both the Pill and IVF, both highly invasive interventions on women's bodies. In the 1980s, both kinds of research are being carried out together: IVF advocates argue that human embryo research must be allowed for, among other things, the development of a 'better' hormonal contraceptive. Such investigations have already been carried out on animal embryos (d'Arcy, 1986).

IVF and hormonal contraceptives are two sides of the same reproductive technology coin. If you drew a family tree of IVF researchers, Pincus would be a parent to today's IVF practitioners. He wrote in the 1960s that his 'work began with a curiosity about mammalian fertilisation and ovum [egg] maintenance' (Pincus, 1965, p. 3). Whence IVF experiments and the Pill. Robert Edwards voiced a similar motivating curiosity: 'I became increasingly fascinated with the *in vitro* maturation of oocytes of various mammals, including man [sic]' (Edwards, 1983a, pp. 53–5). This is what I mean, that women are not a presence in the scientific view of reproduction; only women's body parts are. The processes of pregnancy are relegated to the generic Man's domain, although in fact all members of the human species do not get pregnant. The motivation is the fascination of science.

According to Edwards, in the mid-1960s he and Howard Jones in the USA carried out the 'fundamental work' on egg maturation (ripening the eggs to a final stage in development, so that they may be fertilised) using animal eggs and women's eggs. The first well-documented fertilisation of women's eggs *in vitro* followed in 1970 by physiologist Edwards and his colleague gynaecologist Patrick Steptoe, and his research assistant Jean Purdy. They, therefore, often receive the credit for the first IVF success in history using women's eggs. Reminiscing about that time Edwards said, 'Once again, we achieved major success with human research while the work on animals was insecure' (Ibid., p. 65). Contrary to popular understanding, IVF experimentation on women's body parts was being carried out *alongside* animal experimentation, before the methods were established in other mammals.

Replying to calls in the 1970s by some scientists for preliminary primate studies before IVF was used as a clinical procedure on women, both Edwards and Roger Short in Britain dismissed that necessity. Edwards later wrote in his textbook *Conception in the Human Female* (1980), 'The closest similarities to man are found in the apes and other rare species, which are obviously virtually unobtainable' (p. 668). Whence, we can conclude, experimentation with women for the same purposes. Short said in 1978 that primate studies are too time consuming (Ethics Advisory Board, 1979).

IVF experimentation on women is not admitted to be

experimentation by reproductive technology advocates. There is a false distinction made between laboratory research and clinical practice. Research scientists presume that they are doing 'pure' research, ignoring the fact that women's bodies are necessary for their experimentation in 'human reproduction'. Women in clinical settings have been the experimental subjects of IVF researchers as surely as a female rabbit sitting on their laboratory benches. Human IVF research from the beginning entails experimentation using women, just as experimentation on rabbit eggs or mouse eggs involves the adult experimental animal. The reality is masked by calling experimentation on women 'human embryo research', by calling the setting the clinic instead of the laboratory, and by adapting their style and terms to suit the requirements of medical ethics. Certainly, an embryologist might easily interchange the remarks, 'I need mouse embryos for experiments' and 'I need female mice for experiments'. Certainly, when they apply to funding bodies for grants to support such research, the experiments are duly considered experimentation on animals; the researchers are required to fulfil certain regulations with respect to animals. Embryo experimentation comes under the heading animal experimentation. Yet when it came to using women's eggs, embryos, and other body parts for scientific investigation, the perception of medical scientists was changed.

Many IVF practitioners and scientific bodies, such as the American Fertility Society and the American College of Obstetricians and Gynaecologists, declared IVF to be standard clinical practice by 1984. Yet other scientific articles, and government reports from Ontario, Canada and Victoria, Australia in the mid-1980s conceded that these techniques used on women are *experimental*. They did not, however, go so far to admit explicitly that such experimental techniques being done on women warranted a discussion of the ethics of using women for experimentation.

Acquiring women's eggs was the first problem for IVF researchers who wished to investigate 'human' fertilisation *in vitro*. From the earliest days of his research on women's eggs, Robert Edwards repeatedly mentioned the lack of sufficient numbers of 'human' eggs. In 1980, he reminisced, 'Surely the whole field then was in my grasp – cows, sheep, monkeys – and man, too, if I could only get their eggs?' (Edwards, 1980b, p. 39).

Removing eggs from women's ovaries was eventually perfected

by Patrick Steptoe's adaptation of the laparoscope, an instrument which allows a doctor to observe abdominal organs, in this case women's ovaries. With the addition of an instrument to grab hold of the ovary and another instrument to pull out ripe eggs, laparoscopy has become the most widely used egg-retrieval procedure for applying IVF to women. The early days of laparoscopy were described by Steptoe (1980a, p. 70): 'I discovered how laparoscopy gave a magnificent view inside the female pelvis . . . The difficulty was that the electric lamp became hot quickly or would break so the whole procedure had to be performed very rapidly. It was a smash-and-grab surgical procedure.'

The book in which this quote appears, *A Matter of Life* by Edwards and Steptoe, was written for the public to tell the story of the quest which culminated in the birth of Louise Brown in 1978.[3] I borrowed *A Matter of Life* from the British Lending Library. Next to the above 'smash-and-grab' quote, in the margin someone had scribbled, 'On women's bodies?!'. According to Edwards, in the early days of his work with Steptoe, a journal rejected on ethical grounds a paper the two of them had written about the use of the laparoscope for egg retrieval in women (Edwards, 1983a, p. 59). Those early doubts about the ethics of egg retrieval in women were quickly drowned in the excitement over the scientific feats of IVF, knowledge on the edges of life, as they say.

The eggs Edwards procured in the 1960s, when the problem was simply keeping the eggs alive *in vitro* (outside the woman's body), came initially from women undergoing surgery for gynaecological problems or ectopic pregnancies. By 1970, Edwards and Steptoe were administering fertility drug regimens to women volunteers to boost the numbers of eggs available to the researchers. By the 1980s, not only women on IVF programmes were a source of eggs for IVF researchers; women undergoing tubal sterilisations are also being asked to 'donate' eggs to research projects for developing genetic screening methods on IVF embryos. The Leeds branch of the Women's Reproductive Rights Campaign (1984) has reported that 'the offer of free sterilisation has been used as an incentive for [egg] donation'.

The second problem for the IVF researcher, once women's eggs were in hand, was to show their scientific work as socially useful.

There is much to learn in the published scientific and medical reports of IVF practitioners. Their use of language in their papers on IVF reveals a cover-up: a cover-up of the use of women as the raw material of research science, and the collusion of IVF practitioners with traditional authorities more powerful than themselves. Whether their manipulation of language is deliberate or not, I do not know. The meaning is still the same, however. I use publications by Edwards and Steptoe to illustrate.

Women: from 'Materials and Methods' to 'Patients and Methods'

In 1965, in the prestigious British medical journal, *The Lancet*, Edwards reported his success at keeping eggs alive outside women's bodies. Speaking in the objective language of science, he named eggs (women's body parts) under the heading 'Material and Methods'. Edwards, a reproductive physiologist who had been publishing his work on embryology and genetics for many years, was used to writing for scientific journals, not medical journals such as *The Lancet*. A 'Material and Methods' section routinely appears in scientific papers reporting experimental results. Edwards was presumably in the habit of listing his materials as such. He later adapted his language to suit medical reportage, but awkwardly. In 1970, he published another paper in *The Lancet* this time with his colleague Patrick Steptoe. Here, the heading 'Material and Methods' appeared again, but the material changed from eggs to *patients*. Finally, in their 1983 *Lancet* paper, the heading 'Material and Methods' disappeared. It was replaced with the heading 'Patients and Methods'

Under 'Material and Methods' in the 1965 (p. 926) paper Edwards wrote: 'Ovaries or pieces of ovary removed during operations for various clinical conditions were washed in saline solution . . . The large follicles were dissected out intact, and then punctured into culture medium to liberate the oocytes [eggs] . . . During liberation of the oocytes . . .'. His language of 'liberation' of oocytes is extremely suggestive of the frustration of the IVF practitioner in need of procuring women's eggs for IVF. It certainly betrays a perverse attitude about women's bodies enslaving our eggs, and the role of the scientist-liberator. Elsewhere he similarly talks about 'fluids entrapped within the cumulus cells surrounding the oocyte' (Edwards, 1980a, p. 605).

In the 1965 paper Edwards noted, 'Maturing oocytes provided excellent *material* for cytological [examination of cells] studies' (p. 928, my emphasis). And under the heading 'Discussion' he explained:

> Perhaps the greatest challenges of the present work lie, however, in the prospect of obtaining fertilised human eggs . . . we may shortly be able to obtain numbers of human embryos . . . Indeed, by using priming doses of follicular stimulating hormone it should be possible to obtain many more oocytes per ovary than obtained in the present work. (p. 929)

At this point, Edwards was still in the earliest stages of non-clinical experimentation with women's eggs. So, research requires finding eggs and even giving women-patients fertility drugs so they can donate more eggs. Women finally appeared under the 'Results' section, as patients in a chart detailing their medical problems and the stages of development of the eggs acquired from them. There are no *women* named as the subject of his early research. There are patients with clinical conditions such as 'uterine prolapse'. However, they are not *his* patients. Edwards was at that point a researcher not involved in any way with these women whose eggs he used. A medical doctor with women patients was the go-between.

The IVF patient: from women to couples

In 1970, Edwards, now with Steptoe, reported in *The Lancet* an experiment comparing different hormone regimens on women 'to impose some control over the menstrual cycle and oocyte maturation' (Steptoe and Edwards, 1970, p. 683). They noted relevant findings in rabbit and pig experiments to illustrate the scientific problems they faced. The first entry under 'Materials and Methods' reads: '*Patients* The volunteer patients were the women of infertile married couples numbering forty-six in all' (p. 683). Edwards and Steptoe told these patients [women] that the investigations [experiments] included possible clinical use as infertility treatment. This was a premature assessment of their abilties (the first live birth from IVF did not occur until 1978), and I believe ethically questionable for that reason; but it was a means of acquiring women's eggs for research. It was also a moral necessity. Fertilising human eggs with sperm is a controversial act, much more controversial than just experimenting with women's eggs on their own. You could imagine the public outcry over researchers tinkering with women's eggs and men's sperm in the laboratory out of curiosity and the pursuit of 'pure' knowledge about reproduction. Thus the ultimate aim of IVF research became infertility treatment; and because of the social implications of fertilising women's eggs, a woman attached to a man was thereafter identified as 'egg donor'.

After IVF produced a real baby in 1978, scientific papers began referring to the 'couple' as the patient where previously they had referred only to the single patient (a woman). *Couples* apply for entrance into IVF programmes (e.g. Sher *et al.*, 1984, p. 512); and in Britain *couples* sign the consent form for a woman's medical treatment in IVF programmes (MRC/RCOG VLA Report, 1986). The message is that women don't have babies, couples do. IVF scientists comply: women are not named as going through the manipulations of the researchers, although only women undergo the treatments. Most obviously, Edwards reported in a lecture to the Eugenics Society in London that some of the patients undergoing laparoscopy suffered from oligospermia, a sperm problem in men (Edwards, 1983a, p. 74)! Men do not undergo laparoscopy, women do.

The scientific reports, it should be clear by now, are not 'objective' or neutral as scientists make out, nor even accurate by scientific standards.

The pursuit of women

As I showed above, methods associated with egg maturation and fertilisation *in vitro* were established using women's bodies. By contrast, embryo transfer methods combined with surrogacy, artificial insemination for breeding a better quality offspring, and some methods of sex determination were first played out on laboratory and agricultrural animals. The reasons are obvious. In the early animal work on embryo transfer, before IVF was possible, the embryo came from the pregnant female animal, who was usually sacrificed (as they euphemistically say) during embryo removal.

The scientific methods and technologies used in animal experimentation do not change in the special case of women's reproduction. Artificial insemination, embryo twinning (the splitting in two of an *in vitro* embryo), egg 'donation', embryo 'donation', surrogacy, sex determination, and so on are all techniques of animal husbandry and research on animals, as well as 'infertility treatment' in women.

Edwards once pointed out a difference between animal work and IVF on women:

It must be stressed that this work on patients [women] has no strict parallel in any animal studies, because the oocyte is being aspirated from the mother, fertilised and cultured *in vitro* and then replaced in her, whereas in animals, a recipient female is usually used to carry the fetuses to full term and the donor is discarded. (Edwards, 1980a, p. 696)

This is the difference, the particulars of the disposal of the egg donor?

The aims of using artificial reproduction techniques on animals are to 'find out' what happens inside the female animal and, more practically, to quality control their reproduction. The dairy, cattle and wool industries manipulate animal reproduction in the interests of production. If the health and well-being of the animals are considered at all, it is in the 'best interests of productivity' and the reproductive engineering of offspring with desirable traits. The pursuits of knowledge of 'human reproduction' by IVF is similarly the desire to know and control how women's bodies work. This is for our own good and the good of 'society', we are told.

In vitro techniques first used on animals, such as embryo transfer, were considered applicable to women before the risks or even benefits were known. In his 1965 *Lancet* paper Edwards wrote, 'The transfer of eggs into the uterus via the cervix, a technique which is now *showing promise* in farm animals, would successfully bypass a faulty fallopian tube [in women]' (p. 929, reference removed, my emphasis).

Edwards repeated himself, this time with co-author Steptoe, in the 1970 *Lancet* paper: 'Our initial attempts to transfer oocytes to the oviduct in women have been only partially successful. Alternatively, entry into the abdominal cavity might be avoided by transferring the embryos into the uterus via the cervix, a method yielding *some* success in cattle' (p. 689, my emphasis).

Moreover, the use of similar *in vitro* methods in animals and women is not merely an application from one mammal, say cows, to another, women. The scientific pursuit of women's reproduction is inextricably intermingled in animal experimentation. Edwards once suggested that putting human embryos briefly in sheep or rabbits could be beneficial to learn about human embryo development (Prentice, 1984). In fact he and Howard Jones had inserted women's eggs with men's sperm into the fallopian tubes of rabbits in a study in the 1960s (Edwards *et al.*, 1966, p. 197). In *Conception in the Human Female*, Edwards reported the use of human follicular fluid [which comes from women's ovaries] in early experiments on fertilising rabbit eggs *in vitro* (Edwards, 1980a, p. 606). The alternative method GIFT, developed on women as an alternative to IVF, is now being used on female horses (Vines, 1987).

IVF is becoming more experimental with time, not less. Women in present IVF programmes become the volunteers for various problem-solving experiments aimed at fine-tuning IVF procedures and increasing success rates, in the quest to know everything about the biological processes of women's reproduction. Many different kinds of fertility drug/hormone regimens are used in the various IVF clinics with no consideration of the long-term effects of such powerful intervention on women's health, and no questioning of the disruption of women's healthy life processes. Researchers in many countries are experimenting with women on IVF programmes in their unending attempts at fine-tuning the IVF procedure, or gaining yet another scientific 'fact' about reproduction.

For example, Dr John Yovich's IVF team in Western Australia tried administering the synthetic progesterone Depo Provera to 'subfertile' women on IVF programmes to prevent miscarriage. Despite criticism from many quarters that Depo Provera is known to cause genital tract abnormalities and other health risks, Yovich and company insisted that this kind of hormonal 'support therapy' would decrease 'fetal wastage'[!] in 'subfertile' women (Yovich *et al.*, 1983, p. 711). They added that they would continue to use the drug randomly in a controlled study within their IVF programme.

The most shocking examples of extreme experimentation on women underoing IVF are experiments with the drug Buserelin (or

HOE 766), which is made by the West German pharmaceutical company Hoechst. It is a superactive analogue of the naturally occurring hormone LHRH, leutinising hormone releasing hormone. Buserelin is chemically related to LHRH, but is much more powerful. It is being used on women in IVF programmes in France and Britain to 'blockade' the normal functioning of the woman's pituitary gland. Pretreatment with Buserelin suppresses LH (lutinising hormone) and FSH (follicle stimulating hormone) levels in women whose menstrual rhythm is normal; this allows the IVF practitioner to control follicular growth 'without interference' from the woman's own hormone output (Fleming *et al.*, 1985, p. 197). Françoise Laborie relates that French IVF practitioners explain that the Buserelin acts as a 'chemical pituitary-ectomy' (Laborie, 1987). The pituitary plays a central role in the regulation of the body's hormonal system. Cutting it off chemically is an extreme chemical invasion of a woman's body, a threat to the functioning of other metabolic processes.

The pituitary is connected to another gland, the hypothalamus. These are parts of the brain. The pituitary secretes several hormones which regulate the menstrual cycle, growth and activity of several other endocrine glands (glands which manufacture hormones and secrete them directly into the bloodstream). In turn, the pituitary itself responds to hormone-like substances produced by the hypothalamus, a gland which regulates a wide variety of physiological processes.

Why cut off a woman's normal hormonal functioning? It seems that the spontaneous surge of LH from the pituitary gland in women with normal menstrual rhythm poses two 'problems' for IVF treatment. First, it 'complicates' management of the woman's fertility by the IVF practitioner. Secondly, normal hormonal activity is 'unpredictable', i.e. inconvenient for the hospital staff.

In England, a team including Ian Craft, director of the IVF programme at the Cromwell Hospital in London, reported experiments on two groups of women, both pretreated with Buserelin. One group received the hormone drug HMG, human menopausal gonadotropin, a combination of FSH and LH. The second group received pure LH. The experiment showed that the development of ovarian follicles was similar in both groups of women. From this they were able to gain a little more scientific knowledge, to test 'the hypothesis that the rate and number of follicles developing in the ovary are FSH dependent' (Jacobs *et al.*, 1985, p. 264).

The sixteen authors of the long paper where this experiment, among others, was reported thanked Dr Patrick Magill at the pharmaceutical company Hoechst for supplies of Buserelin, and Dr Ellis Snitcher of Serono for supples of FSH and for financial support.

IVF researchers mine women's bodies. The need for eggs, other body parts, and whole women for reproductive research means the need for a pool of women to become volunteers. The most obvious material example is the pool of women in present IVF programmes. Other women provide raw materials for reproductive research as well, for instance, women undergoing abdominal surgery or sterilisation are potential 'egg donors', birthing women are potential placenta 'donors', women seeking contraceptives are potential 'volunteers' for clinical trails of fertility management products, and women undergoing abortions are potential 'fetus donors', that is we provide the so-called fetal material for research. Women in clinical settings have for decades been providing medical scientists with urine and blood samples, from which hormones and serum for research may be extracted, with cervical fluid, with bits of fallopian tube and uterine tissue.

Many clinical experiments have been conducted on pregnant women since the 1940s. A medical doctor, Maurice Pappworth, chronicaled a series of such experiments in his highly critical book on human experimentation in medical settings, *Human Guinea Pigs: Experimentation on Man* [sic] (1967). One example was the experiments on 181 women in England using cardiac catheterisation when the technique was novel in 1949. Pappworth criticised the experiments on many levels, including the fact that experimenters were unaware of anaemia in at least one woman, and that two separate studies were carried out in two different hospitals – an unnecessary duplication. Another example he gave was the testing of blood-flow in a woman's liver by passing cardiac catheters through her heart into the hepatic vein of the liver in various stages of pregnancy, and there were attempts on two women at full term in their pregnancies. This experiment was performed on fifteen pregnant women altogether, the control being made up of fifteen non-pregnant women who also underwent the same treatment. These are but two examples that Pappworth mentions. Women are the subjects of such experimentation, even when the study is directed at the fetus, and women *always* carry the physical and emotional risks of such experiments and their outcome. Women in clinical settings are not the only captive audience available for reproductive research. For example, prostitutes were used in the 1960s by Seymour Katsh (1969), in the USA, to study immunological aspects of reproduction. Katsch experimented on jailed prostitutes to study the immune response of female to male antigens delivered into the vagina during coitus. Presumably his thinking was that using prostitutes for experiments relating to intercourse was morally acceptable.

The absence of women as women in the realm of scientific inquiry allows this kind of science to proceed. Men too are beginning to come under the knife as scientists 'need' to know about the processes of sperm production increases. However, it is the experimental subordination of the female body that permeates the pursuit of scientific knowledge about reproduction and fundamental life processes. Human embryology and developmental genetics are the study of what goes on in women's bodies.

Human embryology is by definition the study of the developing embryo, or literally, *knowledge* of the developing embryo. That branch of biology ignores the reality that embryology is about *women's* biochemistry and physiology, women's fertility and pregnancy. Women's body parts (egg, placenta, follicular fluid, cervical secretions, wombs) and women's bodily functions (fertility, ovulation, conception, pregnancy) are the objects the human embryologists' first questions.

IVF – the fertilisation of egg and sperm outside the female body and in a laboratory dish – and the maintenance of IVF embryos in the laboratory reduces women's reproductive capacity to that of men: women become gamete donors. This is implicit in the arguments coming from scientists and the scientific establishment to counter the moral disapproval of IVF methods. The recurring arguments are that egg donation is logically the same as sperm donation, that surrogacy is logically the same as artificial insemination by donor, and that genetically a baby is just as much its father's as its mother's.[4]

The different ways of acquiring eggs and sperm and the different processes of sperm donation and carrying a baby to term (baby donation?) are made invisible or reduced to a deceptive genetic statement. Women do not exist in IVF reproduction, rather, parts of the body and women's role as 'gamete donor' are what exist.

For women, yet another impossible distinction is made in the IVF debate, between experimentation and observation, as if the first is manipulation and the second is not. When Robert Edwards was taken to task by the British Medical Association and the British press in the early 1980s for supposedly saying he *experimented* with human embryos, his lawyer explained that in fact Edwards had not 'experimented' with IVF embryos, he 'observed' them (*The Guardian*, 1985). The distinction, of course, rests on who is being manipulated. Women's physical bodies are manipulated (not passively observed) to make IVF embryos from the outset. This is not recognised.

The invisibility of women as the primary subject of human reproduction is apparent in the use of the generic masculine in scientific speech. In scientific writing and speaking, 'man', 'men', 'his' are used to donate human beings generally, as well as the male of the species in particular. Edwards talks about the stages of egg maturation 'in man' (e.g. Edwards, 1965, p. 926). So do most other IVF practitioners, such as Alan Trounson in Australia (Trounson and Conti, 1982). The researcher Henry Leese (1986) used the phrase 'man's eggs' when lecturing on human embryo research at the University of York. This usage is more than just plain weird. The phrase 'man's eggs' to denote eggs taken by intensive invasive procedures on women is a gross insult. We live in a gender divided world. The disappearance of women's unique role in human reproduction is a collective political act, not an accidental scientific bad habit.

When you stop using the word 'man' or 'human' for experimentation and application carried out on women, when you stop naming disembodied body parts like 'man's eggs', the meaning of what is going on changes. Women's presence as experimental subject becomes close, tangible, and obvious. How different it would sound if Edwards wrote *My interest in women's eggs and the possibility of fertilising them outside women's bodies began in the late 1950s*, instead of 'My interest in human oocytes and the possibility of fertilisation *in vitro* began in the late 1950s and early 1960s' (Edwards, 1983a, p. 53).

I am not arguing that the use of reproductive technologies would be less problematic if scientists stopped using the generic masculine. I wish to emphasise the two-faced message of science in the area of reproductive technologies. The terms 'humanity' and 'human reproduction' do not address women as autonomous human subjects, but from the dominant male-defined world view. Despite the statements from scientists that IVF addresses women's needs, their thinking is centred on themselves, what it means for science, and their own brand of human relations. In a presentation to the Eugenics Society in London, in 1982, Edwards could say, 'This decision to replace embryos [in the early 1970s] signalled the onset of a long and frustrating period *for us*' (Edwards, 1983a, p. 66, my emphasis). And

At long last, in 1975, the first successful pregnancy was established...What a wonderful moment! but it ended in disappointment, because it was an ectopic pregnancy, implanted in the oviduct, and the fetus died and had to be removed [i.e., the pregnant women had to be operated on; did she loose that fallopian tube?]. But this was a wonderful stimulus to us, even though the pregnancy ended tragically. We knew that *our* embryos were capable of implanting, that they could attach themselves to the wall of the uterus and were capable of sustained fetal growth. (Edwards, 1983a, pp. 68–9, my emphasis)

Another IVF practitioner, Robert Winston, was also caught out talking about 'my embryos' on British television during a programme exploring the 'ethical dilemmas' of IVF called 'Made in the Lab' (1986).

The nature of reproductive science: technology knowledge

The relationship between science and technology is complex. Each technology has a unique developmental history. The 'problems' scientists (in the broadest sense) see and the questions they pose prompt their inventions of technologies. In turn, technology affects the construction of scientific knowledge. In industrialised culture, this kind of knowledge is considered 'fact', true knowledge, 'better' knowledge. Newspapers report the latest genetic discovery or newest 'test-tube' baby procedure as progress. Even when they criticise the technologies, the situation is portrayed as progress at a price. There is little doubt among mainstream commentators that the technologies themselves reflect an advance in knowledge and human achievement.

In this section I wish to clarify some aspects of the relationship between 'scientific knowledge' about reproduction and the new reproductive technologies, between scientific knowledge and technology knowledge.

In the case of IVF, the problems of science come first. And by the problems of science, I mean more than the particular interests of, say Robert Edwards and present day IVF practitioners. I include the perceived problems of global population control and eugenics, which are concerns of various branches of biological and medical science. I also include the needs of capital, for IVF and related biotechnologies are national and international big business.

Research scientists, or medical scientists, locate women's 'needs' for IVF, and society's 'needs' for scientific reproduction. Though the 'needs' of society are promoted as the aim of IVF research, it is important to understand that the 'needs' of society follow from the technological capability. When IVF practitioner Howard Jones gave evidence to the US Congressional hearing on Human Embryo Transfer in 1984, he 'went on to point out that the process of IVF has *pinpointed several scientific problems,* the solution of which would vastly increase the general understanding of human reproduction and help solve the problem of human infertility' (House of Representatives Hearing Report, 1984, my emphasis).

In vitro methods are perceived by scientists like Robert Edwards as fundamentally necessary to learn about women's reproduction. Knowledge of reproduction depends on the new reproductive technologies. In the words of one researcher, 'In fetal physiology, no less than in other sciences, advancement in the state of our knowledge depends upon the introduction of techniques' (Nixon, 1973, p. 132). From there, the answers IVF give are held as natural truths. IVF knowledge becomes normalised: made normal, as if what IVF practitioners find from their artificial experiments should be accepted by everyone as women's reproductive reality.

We are presented with the scientific knowledge gleaned from experiments as if they are the biological 'facts' of reproduction. An example is Robert Edwards' textbook *Conception in the Human Female* (1980). It is about the processes of reproduction from fertility to implantation of an embryo from about five to twelve days after fertilisation. This book is the scientific interpretation of the first stages of 'human reproduction'. So much of the 'knowledge' is extrapolated from IVF studies on animals and women that the book may well have been entitled 'IVF Conception in the Human Female'. Edwards understands women's fertility against what experimental results tell him. When relevant, he uses *in vitro* practice on animals and women to explain the biological processes of reproduction. He explains, expounds on, and interprets the *in vitro* experiments and clinical practice to shed light on several stages of women's fertility. Techniques such as embryo flushing, embryo freezing, and embryo transfer becomes the basis for understanding implantation, embryo metabolism, and embryo development [i.e. pregnancy]. Yet, these techniques are as far removed from the historic, social experiences of women as they could be. IVF methods are not a mirror of nature. They are reproductive technologies, and are lumbered with all the problems and politics and questionable realities of technology.[5]

Experimental, high-tech invasion of women's bodies is the *modus operandi* of the scientific pursuit of knowledge of reproduction. This scientific approach splits women into two, social-cultural selves who exist, and biological machines driven by physiological processes. The scientific split is necessary for science, and devastating for women. The split would have us believe we are unable to know or control our own reproduction; by it, we should always require an 'expert' whose knowledge is derived from experimenting with women's body parts and whole bodies.

Technology comes at us from both directions. IVF is used to answer questions about reproduction, as in Edwards' textbook on conception; and then IVF becomes the technological alternative to reproduction when 'nature [women] fails'.[6] As I illustrate throughout this book, IVF advocates see innumerable applications of the new reproductive technologies to improve on women's 'faulty' reproduction: not only for women with blocked fallopian tubes, but for genetic selection of embryos, for genetic 'therapy' of embryos, to grow spare parts for medical therapies that have nothing whatsoever to do with reproduction, to test drugs and toxins for their effect on humans, to freeze embryos for later use by couples who are fertile, for sex selection, and more. An aim of the scientific approach is improvement and control. This is not an inference or implication. Improvement and control are *recognised* aims of science.

This means control of families and populations, and most particularly women, as the subjects of the biological processes of reproduction, and as the primary subject for the social control of reproduction. Human reproduction is a social activity, not a reflex biological action. Scientific control *must* mean the social control of women's sexuality and reproduction. Social control of reproduction – of women – is *necessary* to scientific reproduction. In Western countries, this desire to control population is couched in terms of an individual's right to 'choose' reproductive engineering. In a society which comes to expect the scientist–expert to have the right answers and tools, what kind of 'choice' is there for a women who would not like to 'choose' genetic selection of her offspring? There is immense social pressure on women who have doubts to undergo infertility treatment, pregnancy intervention technology such as amniocentesis, and birthing technology.[7]

The need to control socially how women reproduce follows after the scientifically minded mend the split they have constructed between the 'natural' phenomena and social phenomena. The scientific 'facts' about sexuality and reproductive behaviour is at first promoted as ahistoric, biologically based, not culturally based. Then they turn around to say that biological knowledge will favourably inform social norms. Split and mend, according to science.

Scientists, the guardians of 'natural' knowledge, have stepped into politics and the running of society. They presume their social authority, based on their knowledge. The split between 'nature' and 'culture', created by scientists who are very much reflecting patriarchal culture, is mended by scientists when it suits their interests. 'Experts' in women's reproduction are becoming social commentators on sexuality, family relations, women's health care, and quality control of populations. Not because we asked them first, but because they invited themselves into the halls of power, as exemplified by the interest Robert Edwards and other scientists took in defining the ethical and social parameters of IVF and human embryo research.[8]

A renowned scientist working in the field of fetal research, Professor Robert A. McCance, concluded the collection of articles entitled *The Mammalian Fetus in Vitro* with a chapter on the ethical considerations of fetal research. He cited Britain's Abortion Act 1967 and a 1972 government report on the use of fetuses for research. The report recommended that a fetus of over twenty weeks' gestation should be considered viable, and so not a subject for research. McCance disagreed: 'this decision was not in the best interests of society. . .this is the very material on which most valuable work can and should be done' (McCance, 1973, pp. 364–5). By the mid–1980s, IVF researchers were voicing a similar sentiment with respect to the fourteen day limit on human embryo research imposed by the Warnock Committee. The imposed limits, as IVF apologists argued, interfere with research, and are not in the best interests of society.

In *Conception in the Human Female* Edwards commented on the social usefulness of reproductive technologies in the midst of a chapter on experimental findings on the divided mammalian embryo. He offered that human embryos can one day be stored while being 'typed for various characteristics, in a manner similar to studies being carried out on rabbits and cows' (p. 689). Edwards did not give any concrete examples of what he meant. But on the same page he had given one example of studies being carried out on animals: the transporting over long distances and distributing of frozen embryos which are 'unique genotypes or belonging to highly specialized genetic stocks' (p. 689). IVF entrepreneurs in the USA actually have suggested traffic in human embryos (Corea, 1985, pp. 80–1).

The principle of 'scientific freedom' is extremely important to scientists to ensure that they may work with minimum interference from regulatory agencies outside science, and especially the dreaded government intervention.

From the beginning of the public controversy over IVF, the message from IVF practitioners and eventually the British scientific establishment is that laws to regulate IVF are undesirable, and scientists can adequately regulate themselves. They agree that IVF and human embryo research needs some regulation, since the human embryo is a special case. But they require scientific freedom to experiment with human embryos (women) for Progress. In 1971, Edwards co-authored an article with a lawyer, David Sharpe, emphasising the desire for scientific freedom with the usual lack of consideration of the ethics of using women for experimental material. The problem with civil and criminal sanctions, they wrote, is that they all contain an implicit direction, 'ask (someone's) permission before you do your research' (Edwards and Sharpe, 1971, p. 89).

Autonomy of science is deemed particularly important in the area of embryo research because human embryology and its correlative genetics are one of the hottest areas in science today. An editorial in *Nature,* in 1983 (p. 735) said that, among other things the understanding of the course of embryonic development is so great 'that responsibly unfettered research should be wholeheartedly welcome'. They neatly suggested that the scientific establishment could itself set up a formal supervisory group to oversee local ethical committees, and then report back to the public. Scientists would regulate scientists!

Inevitably, we hear the argument that outside regulation of science will herald a new intellectual Dark Age. Time and time again 'scientific freedom' advocates remind us of Galileo (1564-1642), a martyr of Truth, who was silenced by Church authorities because of his (scientifically correct) belief in a sun-centred planetary system. This could happen again, we are told, if scientists, seekers of 'natural' knowledge ('truth'), are supressed in their pursuit of IVF. This analogy is a cheat. The status of scientific inquiry was totally different in the sixteenth and seventeenth century when Galileo lived. Galileo's explanation of the solar system fits observable 'facts'; but the dominant, Church-authorised explanation of an Earth-centred system also fitted common sense observation at that time. More importantly, science today is highly organised; it is an institution, enjoying a great deal of political power and prestige. The Industrial Revolution and two world wars effected a powerful and respected position for science and technology. The interests of individual scientists are well protected by a scientific authority that may well be equal to the authority of the Church in the seventeenth century. Galileo, espousing beliefs at odds with the dominant authority, may have been oppressed. By contrast, scientists in Western, industrialised societies today construct knowledge *within* the dominant, respected belief system, Natural Science, which enjoys funding and support from governments. Scientists are not an oppressed group.

The principle of 'scientific freedom' itself is tempered and qualified within contemporary science. A scientist who depends on funding bodies to pursue expensive, high-tech research is hardly 'free'. In fact the principle of 'scientific freedom' is not about intellectual freedom but about political power: the power of science in society, who controls science, and what science controls.

The journal *Nature,* always defending the cause of science, took the opportunity to make a case for allowing experimentation with human embryos in an editorial entitled 'The Future of the Test-tube Baby'. They expound that human IVF research is a necessary extension of experimentation with animals, and that scientific knowledge of human embryo development is one of the most important questions in science today. As usual, they expressed no appreciation of the fact that they are experimenting on women. They speak about research on 'human embryos' no differently than they would on rabbit embryos:

> The extent to which knowledge of what happens – and what goes wrong – in the early stages of natural embryonic growth can be extrapolated from observations of other than human mammals is strictly limited. Sooner rather than later, it will have to be confirmed with human embryos. And one of the next big prizes in biology, an understanding of the process of differentiation, at this stage sought by observations of laboratory animals, will in due course probably require confirmation in human embryos grown beyond the gastrulation stage (two to two-and-a-half weeks). (*Nature*, 1982)

The Nobel prize-winning experiments are genetic experiments (the 'process of differentiation' is directed by genetic mechanisms). This is the future of the 'test-tube' baby. No 'test-tube' babies, no prize-winning research.

I must emphasise that this 'basic' research on genetic mechanisms exists totally independently of women's health issues. Many research scientists who derive necessary research materials – women's body parts – compliments of IVF have no special professional interest whatsoever in women's health.

Scientists can make a case, if they so choose, that the scientific knowledge of cell differentiation will in future inform clinical medicine and women's reproduction. But they could also make a case for pursuing that line of research for almost *any* health issue. It is not difficult when working on the level of cells (in this case, early human embryos) to construct a relevant scenario. I remember helping with the writing of grant applications to study a cellular mechanism called protein biosynthesis. We sent one grant application to the American Cancer Society and one to the National Institutes of Health. We adapted the ultimate aims and usefulness of the work to suit the funding bodies' interests. And both sets of aims are perfectly credible *scientifically* speaking. Researchers dependent on grants do it all the time.

Genetic questions of 'human reproduction' go beyond the level of the embryo, and genetics permeates the entire field of 'human reproduction', and beyond. The European Medical Research Councils' Advisory Subgroup on Human Reproduction made recommendations in 1984 for priority areas in human reproduction research. It was largely an endorsement of genetic research *of all kinds* on women's body parts and processes. For example, they recommend the use of tropoblasts (cells from placentae) as a human model for the study of gene expression (a 'big prize' project). For another, they recommend research on the adverse effects of environmental toxins which are thought to affect people's reproductive 'performance' or which induce congenital conditions in offspring. They suggest such studies so that 'suitable methods' can be developed for screening individuals at risk of being affected by such toxins. These 'suitable' screening methods come from genetic engineering technology. They were not suggesting removing hazardous toxins from the environment, but screening to locate so-called 'at risk' individuals. Thus the problem is defined, not as the toxin, but as an individual's biology!

Arguing the case for 'human embryo' research to the British public, scientists H. John Evans and Anne McLaren put forward 'practical' projects. They wrote that research on human embryos is necessary (i) to study the 'causes' and mechanisms of infertility, (ii) to circumvent the production and transfer of severely abnormal IVF embryos, (iii) to study the causes of chromosome disorders and genetic defects, (iv) to prevent severe inherited disease in offspring with genetic engineering technology (DNA probes for screening and diagnosis), and (v) to invent better contraceptives.

All these experiments require the use of women's bodies. For that reason alone, they should be considered unacceptable. But having said that, I wish to comment on other problems with these projects.

When they speak about studying 'causes' of infertility and genetic disorders, they mean looking at what goes on at the cellular level. This is not going to be helpful *to women as women*. We already know that a great deal of infertility is preventable, and that a great deal of infertility and congenital conditions stems from poor socio-economic conditions, such as poor nutrition and polluted environments, from doctor prescribed contraceptives, from medical procedures on pregnant and birthing women, from lack of primary health care (see Chapter 4).

Another justification for human embryo research which they put forward, namely to circumvent the production and transfer of severely genetically abnormal IVF embryos, would not be necessary if scientists were not engaged in IVF in the first place. This concern was generated by the existence of IVF; one technology prompts another. From the beginning, IVF practitioners feared that their creation of *in vitro* human embryos would result in abnormal offspring. (By contrast, they accept the accidental and deliberate creation of abnormal or 'monster' (McLaren, 1976) animal offspring from reproductive engineering experiments.)

When discussing the invention of 'better' contraceptives, Evans and McLaren wrote that the ideal hormonal contraceptive could result from research on human gametes (egg and sperm). Such an 'ideal' contraceptive, they explained, would affect only the egg and sperm, but only through *in vitro* experimentation with women's eggs and men's sperm could the risks be ascertained. Women do not need yet another hormonal contraceptive that will affect our eggs, and so the rest of ourselves. We have had enough experience from the ill effects of the Pill, Depo Provera, and other hormonal contraceptives. A contraceptive that is only possible if they remove parts of women's insides to experiment on is not 'ideal'. The 'ideal' contraceptive is one that fits 'ideally' into *their* scientific fertility control thinking, and *their* presumptions about women's sexuality and availability for heterosexual sex. But this new contraceptive is not going to be 'ideal' *for women,* the process of creating it will not be ideal *for women,* and the clinical trials will not be ideal *for women.* Women, most especially women in developing countries will pay the penalties for the 'ideal' hormonal contraceptive. Invasive hormonal contraceptives are 'ideal' for eugenists and other social engineers (Walsh, 1980), and for scientists who wish to follow in the footsteps of Gregory Pincus and other Pill pioneers.

Robert Edwards has added to the list of reasons for growing embryos *in vitro.* For instance, the tissue acquired in this way can be used in transplants and also to treat cancer and diabetes. In other words, women's bodies are needed to produce medical therapies and products for others.

Scenarios of 'practical applications' of 'human embryo' research mask the fact that many of the experimental procedures and technologies originate from 'pure' curiosity about the embryology of mammals and for the purpose of genetic control of offspring. Scenarios about future prospects ('cures' for infertility, 'perfect' contraceptives, and 'perfect' babies) betray a naive trust in science for providing answers for problems that are not merely biological, but inextricably social and economic. Finally, these scenarios are couched in terms of individual benefit, concealing the intent of social engineering.

Part of the allure of pursuing IVF in women is bound up in what scientists perceive as the 'mystery of life' which dwells there. The title of the book which incorporates the British Warnock Report on IVF is *A Question of Life,* not A Question of Infertility Treatment or Women's Health, or even Human Reproduction. Edwards and Steptoe's popular account of their IVF quest on women is entitled *A Matter of Life.* Malestream ethicists and theologians talk about these burning fundamental questions of life. Whereas feminists, and numbers of women active in health care and the birth lobby who would not call themselves feminists, talk in terms of women: IVF and all the reproductive technologies are about women's lives, not a rarefied concept of Life.

I think this aspect of IVF as the key to 'life' is important to understand the extent to which women are exploitable for the pursuit of scientific knowledge. IVF is a key to the scientific question of life, for women's eggs are the quintessential material of life. The much sought after egg, fertilised and developed, is where scientists look for the direct workings of genes in the creation of a living human being. It's heady stuff, human embryology. In an article entitled 'What a Piece of Work is a Man [sic]. . .', Jon Palfreman (1986) considered the science of embryology:

> Life is a remarkable process. . .The biological development of the individual in all the key aspects takes place when we are embryos. . .What then could there be in the first cell [the fertilised egg] powerful enough to co-ordinate this whole process? The answer is genes. . .*The mystery of life then, the big question of biology, is to explain how genes make creatures.* (My emphasis)

IVF as the place to study the mysteries of life holds an extra thrill.

A theme as ancient as history is the myth of the male creator. In Greek mythology it occurs in the story of Athene born from the head of Zeus after he swallowed his pregnant wife, Metis. More subtly, ancient Greek embryology defined the male as the active generative principle of procreation, the women as passive receptacle. This belief continued to inform Western intellectuals up until the twentieth century; it was embodied in a variety of scientific explanations, some from direct observations in nature (now discredited). The image necessitates ignoring women, defining women as less than men, violating women, and destroying women – as in the case of Metis. The image re-occurs in various guises. Mary Shelley told the Enlightenment version as the fictional story of Dr Frankenstein, the scientist who creates a live human being from dead parts, 'I, Victor Frankenstein, had achieved what many men had tried and failed. I had created life!'. Now, IVF and embryo transfer is accomplished by scientists who are called miracle-makers, creators of life; they are called 'test-tube' fathers, not 'test-tube' mothers.

Poet Adrienne Rich wrote in her prose work, *On Lies, Secrets and Silence* that the greatest re-evaluation in a women-centred university will occur in the realm of the sciences. The feminist argument with science and technology is an argument with patriarchy, as surely as are our arguments with the division of labour, with religion, with compulsory heterosexuality, with the nuclear family, with capitalism, with war. Reproductive technology reflects a distinctly Western culture of science and technology. Male-centred reality is as apparent in natural science as it is everywhere else, and the implications are as meaningful. The radical change in the natural sciences that is necessary to ensure a non-exploitative relationship with nature is part and parcel of a similar change in society to relieve exploitation of women in all areas of cultural activity.

The relationship between science and women's oppression is not a question of which came first, the science or the oppression. The problem is that the pursuit of the scientific knowledge of reproduction via *in vitro* studies *requires* the mining of women's bodies. If not, then IVF and the other kinds of studies mentioned in the chapter could not happen in the first place.

6

The new genetics

In 1900, genetics was born when the papers of Austrian botanist Gregor Mendel were rediscovered by scientists thirty four years after their publication.[1] Mendel's observations led him to postulate laws of inheritence to explain similarity and variation in the traits of pea plants and their progeny. Today, genetic considerations have become so much a part of reproductive practice in industrialised countries that it is almost impossible to consider pregnancy and childbirth without them.

There are many practices and rituals which give meaning to kinship and reproduction. The concept derived by scientists, genetics, has become a significant biological 'fact', as if knowledge about genes reflects our experience of inheritance and family ties.

It is important here to realise that modern theories of inheritance were forged in the nineteenth century in Britain and other imperialist countries. Common ideas about the inheritance of intellectual faculties, moral sensibilities, and physical attributes supported ideas about the 'natural superiority' of the white ruling classes and the 'superiority' of the male. These ideas fed into biological theories of inheritance (what became genetics) and evolution. In the late nineteenth century, the word 'eugenics' was coined by the English scientist Francis Galton to denote the science of selective breeding for the improvement of the human 'stock'. Eugenics emerged as an extension of the science of heredity, and then genetics. Theories of inheritance and genetics were (and are) to a great extent dependent on already existing cultural beliefs about sexuality, kinship, gender and racial identity (see Chapter 7).

This chapter is an examination of some genetic technologies

associated with the new reproductive technologies. I wish to overturn the dominant message that genetic knowledge and technology is neutral, and that when applied to 'human reproduction', genetic technology serves women's needs. I wish to challenge the concepts and applications of genetics itself, and what is becoming a genetic ideology in Western societies. I believe that the philosophy and practice of genetics is antithetical to women's health, well-being, integrity and freedom.

The main critical points I wish to make in this chapter are:

1. The growing repertoire of genetic technologies places more physical and psychological burdens on women: more reasons to undergo high-tech, scientist-controlled means of reproducing (IVF, embryo donation, etc.); more invasive testing during pregnancy (fetal surgery, embryo genetic therapy); and more reasons to contemplate for selective abortion of 'afflicted' fetuses. The application of genetic technology is a further medicalisation of women's reproduction.

2. Applying genetic technology to women's reproduction requires the social/biological control of women: the use of women's reproductive bodies for scientifically controlled reproduction, and an imposition of sexist social conditions. Applications such as gene therapy on IVF embryos will be experimentation on women's bodies, and they entail physical risks.

3. Genetic technology is eugenic; it incorporates the thinking that 'better genes make better people'; it perpetuates discrimination of disabled people as more conditions are being diagnosed as 'genetically' based. It identifies some people as 'unfit' because of our genes. It promotes the pursuit of the 'perfect baby'. 'It's as if our children were products and the standards of production have to be maintained', said Barabara Katz Rothman. 'We all have to have perfect babies who can read by age three' (Hopkins, 1985).

4. All the techniques of genetic technology share a common value. They all boil down to the arrogant belief that scientists can identify genes and genetic functions, and that they can control them. This is most apparent in genetic engineering. Yet no one really understands the complexity of genetic mechanisms, and the myriad of other bodily processes that influence the working of genes.

Introducing the new genetics

Today, scientists understand 'genes' as special pieces of DNA, shorthand for the molecule deoxyribonucleic acid.[2] They are present in the cells of our bodies, including egg cells and sperm cells. Genes carry and transmit information from one generation to the next. How is the information transmitted? Each gene contains a 'code' for the manufacture of a specific protein (another kind of molecule). The various proteins in our cells are responsible for body development and functioning. The magazine *Scientific American* encapsulated the role of genes: 'Genes encode proteins, proteins in turn, by means of selective binding, do almost everything else' (1985, p. 3). Whence, the importance biologists place in genes.

Saying genes encode proteins explains the molecular event. What it means is that genes have a basic role in embryo development and life processes such as metabolism. For two examples, eye colour is a genetic (inherited) trait, and insulin production requires information carried by genes.

Today, the language of genetics stresses molecular criteria (genes, 'normal genes', 'faulty genes') for the control of 'human reproduction', that is, which women will breed, with which genes, and how.

The application of genetic technology means that an 'expert' has to make a decision about which genes are good and which are not; which genes should be allowed and which should not. It follows a scientific approach which concentrates on genes, ignoring the sociality of human reproduction, women's subjectivity, the complexities of women's experience of pregnancy and childbirth.

The genetic approach ignores the fact that human reproduction is a social experience, not a 'purely' biological one. For one, the diversity of social and cultural experiences of familial relationships among peoples are made subordinate to the 'norm' of the 'genetic' parent-child relationship. For another, as we all know, birth registrations are not always in accord with the 'genetic facts' of paternity, and perhaps of maternity in a few cases. Putative fathers are not always the 'genetic' fathers; and many couples who use artificial insemination by donor to have children sign birth certificates with the name of the 'social' father.

An example of the imposition of genetic technology on the

social relations of human reproduction is 'DNA fingerprinting', an application of genetic analysis methods used to establish a genetic profile of the subject. In the UK, the government wishes to introduce 'DNA fingerprinting' in immigration cases to 'authenticate' parent–child relationships. The presumption is that only genetically related children are 'authentic' children of a parent.[3] It reduces the fullness of the biological/social experience of parenting where sensuous, bodily acts of love, bonding, and caring for children cannot be reduced to a genetic relationship.

The genetic approach masks in molecular language its eugenic aim. The aim is no longer controlling the quality of the human 'stock'; the contemporary aim is controlling the quality of the human 'gene pool', as they say. This can only be carried out by social control of reproduction.

'Genes' are becoming the criteria of who is fit to breed, who is fit to be born, who is fit to work, and who is fit to live. Genetic technology is a tool of social engineering. Genetic screening of prospective parents identifies adults who are 'carriers' of genetic disease, and who in the language of geneticists pose a 'genetic risk' to the population. Pre-natal screening of fetuses for congenital conditions is carried out by the medical profession with the intention of selective abortion of afflicted fetuses (this is not always women's intention; many women are not certain they will decide to have an abortion after the tests). More recently, the new reproductive technologies have made it possible to analyse the genes of eggs, sperm, IVF embryos, children and adults. And the new technologies have made it possible to alter the genetic make-up of eggs, sperm, embryos, children and adults. The application of genetic technologies on eggs and embryos means, of course, they are being used on women. Beyond their application in reproduction , the new genetic screening technologies may also be used on adults, for example, on prospective employees in the workplace to identify those 'at risk' of ill-health. And according to the most enthusiastic advocates of the reproductive/genetic technologies, they can be used [*on* women, *by* scientists] to direct the course of human evolution (Huxley, 1961a; Grobstein, 1981; Grobstein *et al.*, 1985).

Certainly, one cannot consider artificial reproduction methods, IVF and 'human embryo' experimentation, without considering genetics, genetic technology, genetic selection and genetic engineering. For example, the British Warnock Committee proposed that infertility clinics should be in close working relationship with genetic counselling units. And from the earliest days of debating the use of IVF on women, the new *in vitro* methods were earmarked for treatment of genetic disorders, by IVF practitioners and researchers, by ethical committees, and by government sponsored inquiries (see e.g. Edwards, 1974; Trounson and Conti, 1982; Warnock Report, 1984; Council for Science and Society, 1984).

Genetic ideology

Perhaps the most pointed example of genetic ideology in the making comes from Baroness Mary Warnock, the chair of the British Committee of Inquiry into IVF issues. The Warnock Committee's recommendation for a fourteen day limit on human embryo research set the standard for all research science. How did the committee come up with the fourteen day limit? Mary Warnock explained: 'The genetic composition of the resulting child isn't determined for 14 days. You might say that continuity with your past begins at 14 days. This seems to me to be the important point, rather than when the embryo is alive' (Dunn, 1984).

This is the startling assessment from a philosopher: that our genes give us our human identity. It points up the great influence of scientific knowledge on Western culture.

IVF magnifies the importance of the genetic composition of children. IVF, egg donation, embryo donation, and surrogacy are considered by advocates as better than adoption because all or some of the genetic material comes from the prospective parents. Further, the medical/science/ethical literature often identifies the 'egg donor' women as both the 'genetic mother' and the 'biological mother'. This logic reduces biological motherhood to genetics. Some make that distinction in order to disinherit a 'surrogate mother' who does not provide the egg, but who would carry a pregnancy for another couple from a donated IVF embryo. Thus a women is reduced to the role of an incubator.

The preoccupation with the source of genes supports the high priority being placed on biological paternity. IVF on women is used as a treatment for fertility problems in men. 'Weak' sperm which may otherwise not fertilise an egg in a women's body, may be capable of fertilisation in a laboratory dish (*in vitro*). Australian

IVF practitioner Carl Wood and co-author Ann Westmore offer another variation. They write that it should be possible, based on animal experiments, to inject a women's egg with sperm from a donor to activate fertilisation, and then remove the donor's 'genetic material' and replace it with the husband's sperm (that is, his genetic material) (Wood and Westmore, 1984, p. 117). IVF methods reinforce the prerogative of males to procreate and the use of women's bodies to do so.

A preoccupation with the genetic quality of offspring permeates all aspects of scientific reproduction, not only artificial reproduction techniques. The British clinical geneticist David J. Weatherall called for the integration of clinical genetics into medical school curricula. Weatherall is most famous for his work on the genetics of the thalassaemias – haemoglobin disorders which have a high frequency in Asian and Cypriot populations in Britain.[4] He writes that diseases of inheritance are worse than other diseases because parents feel guilty and responsible, afflicted children are a burden to the community, and marriages break up because of it. Weatherall portrays genetic technology as a 'pastoral' activity of medicine. The 'need' for genetic technology is couched in terms of 'genetic health' versus 'genetic burden' and medicine's priestly role. Weatherall never challenges the nature of the preoccupation with genes and the medical science promise of the 'perfect baby' which create and reinforce feelings of parental guilt.

Where does it end? Ethicists Helga Kuhse and Peter Singer, assistant director and director respectively of the Centre for Human Bioethics at Monash University in Australia, are vocal advocates of IVF technologies, genetic selection of embryos, and now eugenic selection of newborn babies. In *Should the Baby Live* (1985), they rationalise infanticide of children with certain kinds of genetic 'abnormality'. They suggest a time limit of twenty-eight days after birth within which such infanticide might be permitted, based on their belief that up until then infants do not have 'sufficient self-awareness' and so no inherent right to life.

The place of genetics in women's reproduction

The connection between genetics and IVF is straightforward. Human geneticists are interested in IVF technology, and IVF practitioners are interested in genetic technology. For Gregory Pincus, an IVF researcher in the 1930s, 'from genetics to embryology and the study of reproduction was not a mighty step' (Vaughan, 1970, p. 22). Similarly, Robert Edwards' early research was in genetics and embryology; he sustains an interest in the genetics of reproduction, as do many other reproductive physiologists.

Because the fertilised egg contains the information (full set of genes) for growth and development of embryo cells into a complex adult person, the fertilised egg is fundamental to the scientific understanding of human genetics. This is a major reason why research scientists want access to women's reproductive bodies.

One cannot overstate the role of genetic technology in IVF research and practice on women. One of the major questions in the scientific pursuit of women's reproduction is a question of genetics: how is the process of embryo development directed by genes? In other words, how does a fertilised egg with its full complement of genes make a human being? The question is physical and metaphysical. The fertilised egg is considered the material carrier of life. On this 'practical' level, the knowledge of the 'genetic machinery' in embryo development is perceived as absolutely essential for progress in research science and for its application as medical genetics. Beyond the 'practical', the knowledge that comes from the genetics of embryo development is considered by the more philosophical scientists to be knowledge about the mystery of life. In *What Is Life?* (1944), the renowned physicist Erwin Schrödinger instructed biologists to look at the 'aperiodic crystal', genes, to find the fundamental answers to the mystery of life. He likened the life scientists' quest of the gene with the physicists quest of the atom.

Genetic technology is inextricably part of IVF practice. If you reject genetic technology, you reject the most basic scientific questions of IVF.

From the horses' mouths:

(1) The renowned embryologist Conrad H. Waddington (1956, p. vi), one of Robert Edwards' mentors, wrote:

> It seems probable then that the most fundamental embryological theories of the immediate future will be phrased largely in terms of genes. . .no adequate discussion of embryology can be given

without devoting a great deal of attention to the related aspects of genetics.

(2) Clinical geneticist David Weatherall (1984, p. 1141) repeated the message to medical doctors in *The Lancet:*

> Perhaps the most challenging question in human biology is how a single fertilised egg with its 6×10^9 base pairs of DNA [genetic material] turns into a human being.

To pursue these genetic questions, *women's bodies* are needed. Nowhere do these scientists discuss this fact.

Robert Edwards pointed out that work with IVF embryos 'introduces the possibility of genetic engineering or embryological engineering in one form or another' (Edwards, 1980c, p. 187). As the guest speaker at a Eugenics Society Symposium Edwards noted, 'Various manipulations could be carried out on embryos before they are replaced into the mother, and some of these methods could be beneficial' (Edwards, 1983a, p. 100).

The British Warnock Committee accepted the scientific assessment of genetic technology in reproduction. Most of the 'posssible future developments in research' the Warnock Report describes are genetic projects, such as cloning, gene therapy (the euphemism for genetic engineering applied to humans), the use of embryos to test drugs or toxic substances that might damage chromosomes, and embryonic biopsy for the detection of genetic abnormalities in IVF embryos. These projects use women's bodies to answer scientific questions about 'genetic health' and 'genetic risk' and genetic engineering. And although the committee skirted the issue of genetic selection of IVF embryos and cloning, they did not reject the future use of genetic technology for eugenic reproduction.

The Warnock Report was not particularly clear on genetic engineering, certainly not as clear-cut as their endorsement of IVF. They side-stepped the issue of genetic engineering on human embryos by directing the question to the proposed 'licensing authority', authorising them (a number of medical scientists among them) to decide about such matters. In their 1983 memorandum to the Warnock Committee, the English Law Society emphasised the need to control genetic engineering but they left room for future application on IVF embryos (on women) if founded on a 'best interests of the child' test. The Swedish Government Report, *Genetic Integrity,* spoke out against genetic engineering in people, but made an exception of 'gene therapy', that is, genetic engineering for 'medical reasons'. The message we are getting is that genetic engineering is respectable for medical reasons and with respect to legal criteria.

The West German Benda Report on IVF issues banned genetic engineering in human embryos, and in early 1987 the French Government announced a three-year moratorium on genetic manipulations of human genes and chromosomes, and on sexing *in vitro* embryos, because of the eugenic implications. But banning is not the final word on genetic engineering in human embryos. Several IVF practitioners and policy commentators endorse the 'qualified' use of genetic manipulations. Their message is, never say never. In future, the thinking goes, there may be some 'humane' use of cloning and genetic recombination in embryos or gametes, as IVF pioneer Robert Edwards offered on the final pages of *A Matter of Life* (p. 188).

Genetic technologies. . .are a burden on women

Genetic engineering covers a range of techniques aimed at manipulating the genetic composition of living things. There are many applications to women's reproduction. They entail pregnancy manipulation, social control of women and quality control of offspring.

The repertoire of pre-natal genetic diagnostic tests is expanding due to genetic engineering technology. The new 'gene analysis' methods allow direct isolation and identification of 'genes' by medical scientists. Gene analysis multiplies the reasons women should undergo pre-natal diagnostic tests, and provide more reasons to identify a fetus as 'abnormal'. And as Paul Bradish (1987) pointed out, they allow more reasons for the sterilisation of women who are tested as 'carriers' of genetic disease.

Applied to pregnant women, gene analysis allows medical scientists to analyse fetal DNA once the cells are acquired by some kind of pregnancy intervention technology. It may be used to identify disease 'causing' genes with 'gene probes'. For example, in 1987 the gene 'for' a rare form of cleft palate was isolated, and enthusiasts predicted that it may soon be possible to screen fetuses for this condition (McKie, 1987). DNA can be isolated from amniotic fluid cells, the chorionic villi (cells surrounding the fetus in the womb), or fetal blood cells. Cells from IVF embryos could also be used for gene analysis.

Pre-natal disgnosis entails a great deal of time, effort and money to 'find' genes and for screening. A cost-benefits analysis comes into play. According to some proponents of genetic diagnosis, it is cheaper for society to promote selective abortion of 'abnormal' fetuses than to raise handicapped children in the population, and it is better for a women not to have the burden of a handicapped child. Such a policy of negative eugenics is an effort to side-step the social, economic and political commitments which are necessary to support the parents of disabled children, and the social supports necessary to enable the disabled.

Gene analysis makes possible more pervasive genetic screening of pregnant women. Women have begun to voice our doubts about genetic counselling, and many have spoken out about the emotional pain and trauma they have experienced with pre-natal screening technology.[5] Still, more and more genes are being isolated. As of 1985, 3000 single gene disorders had been identified; and over 300 tests are now available for pre-natal diagnosis of metabolic disorders. Some forms of cancer and heart disease are now identified as 'multifactorial' genetic conditions, caused by the interaction of many genes and environmental factors. Extending the genetic hypothesis, as the geneticist Victor McKusick did in 1964, *all* disease has a 'genetic component' (McKusick, 1964).

Genetic technology changes the understanding of cause: genes become the cause. Genetic analysis of fetuses is perceived by its advocates as 'preventative medicine' (Newmark, 1986). In the gene-centred approach to reproduction, 'preventative medicine' means identification of a congenital condition such as cleft palate. It places burdens on women to make eugenic decisions about abortion and about risky interventions such as 'fetal surgery'. By contrast, in a women-centred approach, preventative medicine means securing adequate primary health care, adequate nutrition, and other social, economic, and environmental conditions for the health of women in the first place. (This medical/scientific approach to genes-as-the-cause is similar to the rationale behind the promotion of IVF as a cure for infertility-the-cause. As I discuss in Chapter 4, instead of addressing known causes of infertility (infection, environmental pollution, IUDs, and so on), the British Warnock Inquiry named infertility a *primary cause* of a medical problem, and IVF a proper cure.)

One genetic technology directed at women's reproduction prompts yet another. Pre-natal screening may now be accomplished in women by a relatively new pre-natal test, chorionic villi sampling (CVS). CVS is being considered as an alternative to amniocentesis. Chorionic villi are tissue surrounding the fetus which originate from the fertilised egg; thus the villi cells have the genetic make-up of the fetus. A doctor locates the villi tissue with ultrasound and removes it with an instrument inserted into the women's vagina, through her cervix and into her uterus (in a variation of this procedure, a needle is inserted through the pregnant women's abdomen and womb in order to remove the tissue). CVS is carried out between eight to twelve weeks of pregnancy, while amniocentesis cannot be carried out until sixteen to eighteen weeks. Thus, CVS allows doctors to diagnose genetic disease much earlier than by amniocentesis. It is experimental and carries risks; it's safety has yet to be determined; and possible errors in diagnosis are higher than in amniocentesis (See Hogge *et al.*, 1986; Elias *et al.*, 1986; Ridler and Grewal, 1984).

Proponents point out that CVS allows earlier eugenic abortion, which might be less traumatic for the woman. However, there is another reason CVS is considered better than amniocentesis. CVS could allow doctors to locate a fetal 'abnormality' early enough for fetal surgery, including gene therapy (altering the genes). Already, surgical repair work is being tried out for neural tube defects and spina bifida in fetuses. A US cytogeneticist John Wiley expanded, 'In the very near future *in utero* [on women] correction of various genetic anomalies may be possible' (*Ob Gyn News*, 1985b). For this reason, gene therapy, Wiley argued a case for using CVS.

Genetic screening was invented by eugenists, and its social control aspects have been apparent since the 1960s (e.g. see Hubbard, 1985; Kevles, 1985). The vast potential of genetic screening with new technology takes the social control capability further. It is in the interests of society, we hear, to set up centralised registries of people who carry major genetic disease. No doubt this kind of registry will place a tremendous social burden on certain women *not* to reproduce, or to undergo genetic analysis, or IVF with egg donation, or fetal surgery during pregnancy.

It is most important to recognise the variety of inherited

abnormalities that scientists identify, and that a great many congenital conditions are *not* inherited. A vast amount of health problems in newborns are caused by 'random mutations' (chance occurance of damaged genes), by environmental factors (e.g. industrial pollutants such as dioxin or 'low level' nuclear radiations), by medical interventions during pregnancy and childbirth, by hazardous working conditions which damage the reproductive systems of women and men, and so on. Paula Bradish found from her examination of genetic counselling in West Germany that the distinction between genetic (inherited) and other kinds of congenital conditions is not clearly made in much of the literature espousing genetic screening of pregnant women. In some cases, the literature makes inherited conditions appear more prevalent than they actually are (Bradish, 1987).

Genetic technology allows population quality control instead of social change. You don't have to demand higher environmental safety standards from industries if you have genetic technology; instead, you screen for people who are 'susceptible' to the particular toxins of those industries.[6] You don't have to worry about poor living and health standards among women, or reproductive hazards in the workplaces of women and men; instead, you just screen for damaged fetuses, and then abort or genetically 'fix' them. You don't have to worry about discrimination against those disabled in ways society will not accept; instead, you just engineer the removal of certain kinds of people from the population. Gene analysis is an approach which eliminates the need for changing repressive economic and political conditions. And as the disability rights movement stresses, the message that this eugenic tactic relieves suffering is bogus, since most handicap in the population is not of genetic origin, but occurs after birth, from accidents and disease. Discrimination and lack of support systems contribute to the disability of the disabled.

Pregnancy manipulation

IVF allows medical scientists to manipulate embryos. Two prospects already accomplished in laboratory animals and agricultural animals are cloning methods called 'nucleus substitution' and 'embryo division'.

In nucleus substitution the nucleus inside an unfertilised egg cell is destroyed and replaced with a new nucleus taken from a donor cell. The nucleus of a cell contains the genetic material; the new nucleus, then, replaces the 'genes' in the egg with the 'genes' of the organism from which the donor cell was taken. Since the replacement nucleus is taken from a cell which contains a full complement of chromosomes (unfertilised eggs contain only half the full complement), the egg may then begin to develop as if it were fertilised. Several researchers have suggested that this procedure could be used with women's eggs to grow genetically specific tissue or organs for transplants, that is for using women's eggs to create medical products for someone else's therapy.

'Embryo division' or 'embryo twinning' is making several/two animals with exactly the same genetic make-up. When a fertilised egg begins to divide, the resulting cells are identical. At the earliest stages of cell division, each cell has the potential to grow into an adult. An IVF embryo can be split in two at this early stage; and identical twins result. This kind of cloning could be used on human IVF embryos at the four-cell stage. After the cells begin to differentiate, twinning is not possible. Embryo twinning is used on cows and other animals for commercial breeding.

Both Robert Edwards in England and Carl Wood in Australia propose that inserting twinned embryos in a woman's womb might increase the success rates of IVF. They see this high-tech intervention in a woman's pregnancy, and all that it means physically and emotionally for women, as similar to what goes on in an ordinary pregnancy. Wood and co-author Ann Westmore wrote, 'By *copying nature* – using microsurgery – the chances of conception and twins could be increased in infertile couples' (Wood and Westmore, 1984, p. 115, my emphasis). Edwards told the Eugenics Society that he finds embryo twinning ethically acceptable since human twins occur in normal pregnancies. Human embryos could, in principle, be split in four and this possibility, Edwards (1983a) believes, is ethically problematic.

Edwards suggests another reason for human embryo twinning. One embryo could be tested for chromosomal abnormality so that a (eugenic) decision can be made whether to insert its twin into the woman's womb. The sex of the embryo can be determined by chromosome analysis of a twin, and could be used where there is a risk of sex-linked genetic disease; only correct-sex embryos would be inserted into a woman's womb (Ibid.). He does not explain how the typing of one twin embryo fits into his rationale that twinning happens-in-nature. Used as Edwards suggests, embryo twinning is a form of negative eugenics, decreasing the propagation of the genetically 'unfit'.

Embryo division might also be used to attempt to create offspring with 'superior' traits. It is already being tried in animal husbandry to create offspring with traits inherited from several parents, by using techniques of splitting and then fusing embryo cells from three or more 'thoroughbred' parents.

Embryo twinning is not the only way scientists can analyse the chromosomes and genes of an IVF embryo. In mammals, a cell from an early embryo can be removed and examined while the embryo, if it survives the operation, can be inserted into a female's womb and a pregnancy result.

IVF practitioners worldwide believe that pre-insertion sex tests and genetic analysis could be carried out in embryos. Carl Wood suggested that sexing of IVF embryos might be the preferred approach to reproduction by parents who are carriers of X-linked genetic disease, instead of amniocentesis and selective abortion of male fetuses. (Some inherited disorders are sex-linked, which means the 'faulty' gene problem occurs on the sex chromosomes. There are two sex chromosomes, called X and Y. Most sex-linked disorders affect males, such as haemophilia. See glossary.)

Now, sex selection of IVF embryos is possible. In June 1987, two IVF teams in Britain, Robert Winston's at the Hammersmith Hospital in London and David T. Baird's at the University of Edinburgh, succeeded in identifying the sex and detecting hereditary genetic diseases in IVF embryos, which is called 'preimplantation diagnosis' (*The Guardian*, 1987b; Johnston, 1987). The University of Edinburgh team is using a 'gene probe' method to identify the Y chromosomes in four to eight day old embryos. The method could also be used on embryos conceived in a woman's body which is flushed out of her womb before implantation. In the national newspaper *The Guardian* Andrew Veitch reported: 'Couples who know that they risk passing on genetic defects such as muscular dystrophy, haemophilia, and some forms of mental deficiency, will be able to use test-tube baby techniques to choose healthy children' (Veitch, 1987b). Both groups said it would be unethical to use the method to choose for a preferred sex, but one of the pioneers, Dr John West, admitted, 'we couldn't prevent the technique being used that way' (Johnston, 1987).

Sex-determination after conception is one approach to sex-selection of embryos and fetuses. Sex-predetermination methods are the latest possibility in sex engineering, where the desired sex of the offspring is orchestrated during conception. Several methods are feasible. One approach takes advantage of the fact that sex is determined by sperm, some of which are male-producing and some of which are female-producing. The procedure entails separating the sperm, and then using either the male-producing sperm or the female-producing sperm with artificial insemination or IVF. Medical scientists insist that this method would be useful in relation to X-linked disorders, to avoid producing male offspring for couples who might possibly pass on such a disorder. However, there is much more interest and research in sex-determination technology than is warranted for such a limited application (see Corea, 1985; Corea *et al.*, 1985; Hopkins, 1985).

Obviously all forms of sex-selection technology may be used to choose for a preferred sex in offspring. Some advocates of sex-selection technology, most evident in the USA, go as far to say that 'sex choice' is a reproductive right of parents. In her article 'High Tech Pregnancies' (1985), Ellen Hopkins gives a critical whirlwind tour of present and future prospects in pregnancy intervention technology. She quotes Dr Ronald Ericsson, president of a biotechnology firm in the USA, who claims to have a sex-preselection procedure for seperating girl-producing sperm from boy-producing sperm. 'Hell', he said, 'if the world doesn't go the way you want it, why not use it?'. His technique was being tested in thirty-eight clinics worldwide as a sex-choice procedure (*Hospitals*, 1985).

The implications of sex-predetermination are depressingly apparant in a study by Roberta Steinbacher and Becky Holmes (1985), which shows that young North American men and women who consider themselves sensitive to female inequality would still choose to have male babies if sex-predetermination technology were available to them. Sex-predetermination, or sex-determination with IVF, would allow couples in Western cultures to choose the preferred (usually male) sex without the stigma that would be attached to using amniocentesis or CVS with selective abortion.

In 1986, doctors at the Fertility Institute of New Orleans announced the first known birth of child by a combination of sex-predetermination and IVF. It was a boy, the result of fertilisation *in vitro* using the mother's egg and the father's male-producing sperm. Details have not been readily forthcoming about this IVF/sex determination conception, but it is obviously not a case of using the technology to by-pass conception of male offspring 'at risk' of X-linked disease.

Sex-choice technology undermines women's struggle for equality. In 'The Continuing Deficit of Women in India and the Impact of Amniocentesis' (1985), Madhu Kishwar exposes the bias built into Western technologies. She points to the failed 'Green Revolution', the mechanisation of agriculture in rural parts of India, as bringing about a further devaluation of women. Women in these areas lost their role as cultivators, their economic status and their livelihoods, as men took over their work with mechanisation. She compares the disinheritance of these Indian women with another 'technical fix', the spread in India of using amniocentesis with selective abortion of female offspring for sex-choice.

Speculating on a future when sex choice could be a reproductive option of couples, Robert Edwards noted, 'Imbalance of the sexes could probably be prevented by recording the sex of newborn children, and adjusting the choice open to parents' (Edwards, 1974, p.12). His is a revealing statement of sex choice possibilities and the state/scientist control of that reproductive 'choice'.

Gene manipulation. . .is a burden on women

When medical scientists refer to the 'new genetics', they mean the use of 'gene manipulation' methods, a specific kind of genetic engineering technology. These methods are considered the most powerful tools for genetic engineering to date. They are so important to science and industry that the term 'genetic engineering' is often used interchangeably with 'gene manipulation'. Such methods are the key to the proclaimed 'age of biotechnology', the exploitation of biological sources and technologies to create products for industry, for medicine, and for the military. Gene manipulation methods are the basis of the new pre-natal diagnostic tests by 'gene analysis', of which I spoke above.

These techniques involve the isolation, identification and manipulation of individual genes. Never before has genetic engineering occurred so directly. Embryo twinning, nucleus substitution, and sex-predetermination methods occur on the cellular level. Gene manipulation occurs on the molecular level, on the level of the genes which dwell in the cell. The basic techniques are known as 'recombinent DNA' technology.

Gene manipulation is used in research science to find out about genetic mechanisms and to control genetic processes. The methods have been applied to everything that carries genetic material – plants, animals, bacteria, viruses, and more esoteric entities like plasmids (pieces of DNA not associated with chromosomes) and rickettsia (a micro-organism). Gene manipulation is directed at a host of medical applications, from genetic diagnostic screening and gene analysis, to gene therapy and vaccines.

Once a gene is isolated using recombinant DNA methods, it may be transferred into the DNA of an organism. 'Gene transfer' has already been accomplished in bacteria, viruses, plants, and animals. For use in humans, gene transfer is called 'gene therapy' or 'gene replacement therapy'.

'Gene therapy' is defined by the US medical scientist W. French Anderson (1984, p. 401) as 'the insertion into an organism of a normal gene which then corrects a genetic defect'. Gene therapy can be directed at the level of eggs, embryos, fetuses, children and adults.

Carl Wood and the IVF policy 'expert' Clifford Grobstein suggest that gene transfer in IVF embryos is a future prospect in gene therapy. From Australia, Dr Ron Trent expects the use of gene manipulation in embryos by the 1990s (Harris, 1985). Gene therapy on eggs, fertilised eggs and IVF embryos is first and foremost experimentation on women. Applying it to humans means applying it to women. It means more IVF experimentation on more women.

Just as *in vitro* methods were first done on laboratory and agricultural animals, likewise with gene transfer. Experiments on mice and rabbits presage similar possibilities on women's eggs and IVF embryos. Gene transfer experiments have been carried out on fertilised eggs of mice, pigs, sheep, and rabbits. Among other researchers around the world, Ralph Brinster and Robert Hammer's group in the USA pioneered experiments on mouse eggs in the early 1980s. They established methods for microinjection of rat growth hormone genes (and human growth hormones genes) into the eggs of dwarf mice. The mice are called 'transgenic' because they carry working genes from another species (in this case rat or human).

In 1984, Brinster's group announced the 'partial correction' of a growth disorder in mice by manipulation of the genes in egg cells. They inserted the gene for rat growth hormone into mouse eggs *in vitro*. Some of the offspring grew, but to one and a half times the size of normal mice. Other malformations and health problems appeared in the giant mice, and the female offspring were infertile (Hammer *et al.*, 1984). The experiment illustrates an obvious problem with the technical approach. Although researchers are clever at isolating and transferring genes, they do not know enough about, and how to control, the cascade of genetic mechanisms. 'The problem,' admitted David Weatherall (1985, p. 154), 'is that we have only the haziest ideas about how genes are regulated in higher organisms'.

The Brinster and Hammer group suggested that transgenic mouse strains should provide useful animal models for the study of several types of human growth disorder (Hammer *et al.*, 1985a). To take these experiments to the human level means more women must reproduce by IVF. It also makes one wonder about their suggestion that human growth disorders be studied in this way.

Genetic engineering of embryos and fetuses, touted by advocates of genetic technology as a medical therapy, is yet another imposition on women's reproduction by medical science. It is more of the same medicalised approach to reproduction: drastic measures for new conditions created by medical scientists with genetic technology. It is yet another imposition on the disabled, an expansion of the meaning of 'genetic abnormality' as something that should be 'fixed'. Gene therapy promotes 'genes-the-cause' with no consideration of the obvious questions about 'normality' and 'abnormality', and then concepts of 'illness' and 'disease'. And especially with no consideration that the 'technical fix' (ultrasound, amniocentesis, CVS, selective abortion, gene therapy, fetal surgery, etc.) for the 'causal' genes happens on women's bodies.

The age of biotechnology

I have not touched on many allied applications of genetic engineering in industry to make products such as insulin and human growth hormone, and by the military to create biological weapons (see Bullard, 1987), or on the social control implications of 'DNA fingerprinting' (DNA analysis), which is being used in Britain and elsewhere to identify individuals in police work (*The Guardian*, 1987a; Newmark, 1987). Nor have I explored the commercial aspects of agricultural and biomedical applications. One example is the 1987 decision by the US Patent Office allowing the patenting of genetically engineered animals. Never before had they permitted patenting of living things. And although the patenting of human beings is forbidden, an unnamed US Patent Office official was quoted as saying that, in future, the rules could be revised to include the patenting of new human characteristics (BBC Radio 4, 10 September 1987). For another example, at the 1987 meeting of the British Association, Dr Michael Hall of the pharmaceutical company Roche suggested that the genetic engineering methods being used in the development of vaccines against the disease *AIDS* had wider implications. He was quoted, 'It would mean that we could manipulate at will the genetic pool, produce super races, modify ethnic traits, excise socially-unacceptable habits – in fact produce people to order' (*The Guardian*, 1987c).

All these applications of genetic engineering are relevant to a discussion of the new genetics of reproduction, for they are all part of the age of biotechnology. They all share the same techniques *and the same values.*

This is the crux of my argument with genetic engineering: the link among all applications of genetic engineering is not a mere sharing of certain 'technical' techniques. The technology carries its conceptual baggage to all areas. Biotechnology boils down to the arrogant belief that scientists can identify genes, reorder them, manipulate them, and control genetic mechanisms. It carries grave risks, and entails social/technological control of all living things. The applications of biotechnologies of reproduction go much further than any previous attempts by state institutions to control nature and women technically.

The philosophy behind biotechnology is that the technology will enhance the quality of life. Genetic engineering will supposedly bring better crops, better pesticides, better medicines, better farm animals, better people, better weapons, and a better approach to women's reproduction. 'Unimagined fields will emanate', waxed the UK's Science and Engineering Research Council (SERC, 1986).

But, the genetic engineering approach itself takes no account of the complexity of living things. First, it promotes technical solutions for economic and social situations. For example, human growth hormone created by genetic engineering methods is being promoted as a 'cosmetic drug', like plastic surgery, one point being that it is socially advantageous to be tall (Davies, 1987). And second, the genetic engineering approach carries untold risks and hazards. The most obvious example is the release of genetically engineered organisms into the environment, which has already happened in the US; such releases are potentially ecologically disastrous. [7]

Yet countries all over the world are embracing the new developments and capabilities in biotechnology.[8] As a booming Western growth industry, biotechnology is touted as a stimulus to the current world recession, the depression of chemical and engineering industries, and the energy crisis. For the West, this translates to more profits for big companies, more markets, more products for consumption, ever more supplies for high-tech medicine, and the death knell to small farming and dairy enterprises.

For 'Third World' countries, biotechnology is sold as a boost to development. Medical scientists argue that the use of genetic engineering in developing countries will contribute to prevention of genetic disease, vaccines and diagnostic agents for parasitic and infectious diseases, and for improving the world food supply. These promises ring hollow against the reality of racist population control policies, racist development programmes which benefit Western industry, the dumping of dangerous medical products by pharmaceutical companies (remember the nursing formula scandal[9]), and the lessons learned from experiments with mechanised agriculture. To promote *the development of people,* biotechnology is not the answer, inded it is a hindrance. For one example, as of 1986, 66 per cent of the population of Guatemala had no access to health care. The Guatemala Committee for Human Rights (GCHR, 1987) estimates that 70 per cent of infectious disease which brings child death could be alleviated with basic community health care facilities.

The promises of genetic health and better products hide the lies, the uncertainties, and the costs which women incur in the implementation by medical scientists of their new genetic technologies of reproduction. They are eugenic, and as they are

Beyond Conception

being applied to all living things, pose great danger to all of nature and to the social welfare of all people.

In an article entitled, 'Engineering a Molecular Nightmare' (1987), Erwin Chargaff, famous for his instrumental work in the 1940s which informed later discoveries about DNA, wrote a powerful statement against the path along which research is being carried out in the field of human reproduction. An Austrian biochemist, Chargaff was forced to leave Europe when the Nazis rose to power. With the splitting of the atomic nucleus and the manipulation of the cellular nucleus (heredity), he wrote, 'Science is now the craft of the manipulation, modification, substitution and deflection of the forces of nature.' He went on to say:

Helping a few couples condemned [sic] to childlessness towards getting a child may strike the obstetrical cytologist as such a laudable step, but we can already see the beginning of human husbandry, of industrial breeding factories. . .I think society could prevent all that and more, but I fear it will not. What I see coming is a gigantic slaughterhouse, a molecular Auschwitz, in which valuable enzymes, hormones and so on will be extracted instead of gold teeth. (p. 200)

Patricia Spallone

7

The new eugenics

> Eugenics is the political arm of genetics.
> (Medawar and Medawar, 1977, p. 56)

Eugenics is the science of 'improving' the human species, or the science of selective breeding. It was a nineteenth-century innovation of scientists and others concerned with the influences of heredity on human characteristics and behaviour. By the turn of the century scientists recognised 'primary functional units of heredity': genes. Thus the science of genetics became the scientific basis of twentieth-century eugenics. Eugenists used theories of heredity and then genetics to 'prove' that mental characteristics and behaviour which deviated from the 'norm' were hereditary.

Eugenists today, like their forebears, are concerned with the genetics of human behaviour in its widest sense, including the 'genetic basis' of disease. The domain of eugenics is grand: it's subject matter encompasses life to death. Eugenists address the social and genetic influences on fertility and childbirth, motherhood, the family, the relationship between heredity and behaviour, heredity and physical traits, heredity and health, and the effects of environment and social factors. In other words, eugenics presumes to encompass all human existence. Eugenists include natural scientists, social scientists, ethicists, medical authorities, policymakers, theologians, politicians, law-makers – professionals whose interests are served by eugenics.[1]

In this chapter I explore one particular aspect of eugenics: how science and technology bears on it. This is mostly a look at the

133

intellectual underpinnings of eugenics and the accountability of scientists creating eugenic knowledge and practice. I contest the mainstream assessment of the global 'population problem', as a construction of eugenics, and show how the philosophy and practice of eugenics today, like the 'old' eugenics, is racist, ableist, and sexist.

The 'old' eugenics . . . the 'new' eugenics

Based on the theory of eugenics are horrific practices. Eugenics is a dumping ground for racial, sexual and class prejudice. The eugenics movement extended already existing social control and punishment of the poor, the 'feebleminded', the less able bodied in the population, and others identified as 'inferior'.

Many social activists from every political persuassion embraced eugenics. One example is the philosopher Bertrand Russell, who is respected today for his activism in the peace movement. In his 1929 book *Marriage and Morals,* he criticised 'a quite exceptional lot of nonsense written on the subject of eugenics' but went on to expose his own eugenic feelings,

> Feeble-minded women, as everyone knows, are apt to enormous numbers of illegitimate children, all, as a rule, wholly worthless to the community. These women would themselves be happier if they were sterilised, since it is not from any philoprogenitive impulse that they became pregnant [?!]. The same thing, of course, applies to feeble-minded men. There are, it is true, grave dangers in the system . . . These dangers, however, are probably worth incurring, since it is quite clear that the number of idiots, imbeciles, and feeble-minded could, by such measures be enormously diminished. (Russell, 1985, p. 167)

Eugenics lost its prestige among many social activists by the 1930s and 1940s when many of its abuses became alarmingly apparent. The most publicised of these were sterilisation laws in several countries and Hitler's euthanasia programme under the Nazi regime in Germany. Compulsory sterilisation laws were enacted in some of the United States in the 1920s, and in Sweden, Denmark, Finland, and Switzerland to curb procreation of certain kinds of people, mostly the poor, Blacks and Native Americans in the USA, and the institutionalised. Britain never had a sterilisation law. Only one eugenics law as such existed here, where eugenic policy was more often implemented indirectly (Davin, 1978; Kevles, 1985). 'Racial hygiene', a concept formulated by eugenists, became the basis of Nazi political philosophy and was the justification for a sterilisation law in 1933 which grew into a genocide law. The Nazi eugenics programme was directed primarily against Jews, and also gypsies, lesbians and gay men, and others considered biologically (racially) 'inferior': those considered 'inferior' were sterilised, used for atrocious 'medical' experiments, tortured and exterminated. Despite its appalling consequences, eugenics was never abandoned by science.

There have always been scientists in good standing, among the scientific élite, who promote eugenics, such as Francis Crick who was awarded the Nobel prize for the co-discovery of the molecular structure of DNA, and Julian Huxley, the first director general of UNESCO (see Corea, 1985 and Kevles, 1985 for the eugenic work of these scientists and others). Both Crick and Huxley offered suggestions for eugenic breeding programmes, presuming that scientists can make decisions about whose genes should be propagated and who is 'fit' to breed.

Eugenics is not a hobby of a few 'misguided' scientists. The Eugenics Society in London, founded in 1907 as the Eugenics Education Society, still exists. Scientists of excellent repute have taken part in its activities all along. According to its 'Aims and Activities' leaflet, in the 1980s the Eugenics Society is a charity which promotes and supports scientific research of eugenic interest. Reputable geneticists and biologists continually appear as speakers at the annual two-day symposia. The new reproductive and genetic technologies are among the most visible concerns of the Eugenics Society (e.g. Benjamin *et al.* (eds), 1974 and Carter (ed.), 1983a).

The new reproductive technologies compel a new eugenics.[2] IVF pioneer Robert Edwards delivered the keynote Galton Lecture, named after the nineteenth-century champion of eugenics Francis Galton, to the Eugenics Society Symposium in London, in 1982. He placed the new reproductive technologies among the tools of eugenics, saying, 'The primary ethic is clear. Any child born after a conception *in vitro* must be normal, and delivered into a loving family' (Edwards, 1983a, p. 94).

At the same symposium, Cedric Carter, director of the Medical Research Council Clinical Genetics Unit, extended the eugenic use of the new reproductive technologies (NRTs). He stated that the technologies must mainly be utilised by parents who already have two children, to 'balance' their use by the infertile and the genetically handicapped. In other words, reproductive technologies for all women. The reason presumably is that he feels it would be detrimental to a eugenic plan if infertile couples (not intrinsically 'good stock'?) and the genetically handicapped (also not intrinsically 'good stock'?) procreate with technology while the 'better' genes of the population lag behind. Carter (1983c, p. 209) also commented that human cloning has an obvious 'advantage' in that it short-circuits the 'lottery' of random chromosomal segregation. (To explain the thinking behind Carter's comment, chromosomes are the structures where genes are packaged in the cells. Each human being inherits half its chromosomes from the mother's egg and half from the father's sperm. Thus each person is a unique genetic mixture. By contrast, a human clone would be genetically identical to a single individual. A clone is produced by asexual reproduction, that is without the union of egg and sperm.)

The resurgence of eugenics as a contemporary theme in biology stems largely from advances in the NRTs. Artificial reproduction technologies have become a social pressure for public acceptance of the so-called 'new' eugenics.

Commenting on the implications of IVF technology the journal *Nature* predicted and endorsed the public return of eugenics:

> If at some point it becomes common that in the course of avoiding genetic defect, some parents also seek to improve on what their own genes would produce, there may be great resentment among potential parents to whom these opportunities do not occur, or are denied. Yet in principle, there can be no persisting objection to constructive eugenic practices provided that they do not weaken the ties that normally bind parents to their children (one generation to the next). No doubt this is the agenda for the next [government] committee on this kind of subject. (*Nature*, 1984)

This quote sums up two allied concerns of eugenics: 'improving' the genetic stock while preserving prevailing family relations. Female reproductive and sexual autonomy impedes this plan, for if women are truly autonomous, then medical/scientific authority loses its élite status and control in the area of reproduction.

Eugenics and the ideology of motherhood

Eugenic breeding programmes have historically depended on the subordination of women as a group to the ideals of home and family. For this end, women's motherhood has been defined from the outside, by 'experts'. From its beginnings, the task of 'improving the racial stock' was deemed a matter of both heredity and rearing, especially a matter of motherhood.

In her immensely valuable article, 'Imperialism and Motherhood' (1978), historian Anna Davin delineates the construction of an ideology of motherhood forged for the service of the British Empire at the turn of the century, to propagate a 'virile race, either of soldiers or of citizens'(p. 16). Motherhood was defined as self-sacrificing womanhood, where extended kinship ties were considered dangerous to the well-being of children. Parenting, especially mothering, could no longer be left to individuals. A social welfare system was seen as necessary to mould mothering and the family. Socialists as well as conservatives supported the ideology of motherhood, all for the good of the nation. The primary agents of control of motherhood were health and social welfare 'experts',especially doctors, their assistants, and eugenists.

For the good of the nation – times haven't changed. Cedric Carter, a fellow of several genetic societies and the Eugenics Society, has repeatedly stressed the primacy of the nuclear family (Carter, 1968, 1983b). At the 1982 Eugenics Society symposium on the NRTs Carter said: 'Our genus, *Homo*, has, I believe, evolved over the last two million or so years using as the main reproductive unit the nuclear family of father and mother, strongly pair-bonded, and their children' (Carter, 1983c, p. 211). Carter warned against disrupting the patriarchal social order; he slips the nuclear family into the realm of the 'natural': some family units are better than others for evolutionary (survival) reasons.

Where there is good motherhood, there is bad motherhood. At the 1967 Eugenics Society Symposium, Carter extended a discussion of screening of male babies with an odd XYY chromosome pattern (instead of an XY pattern which occurs in most males). The XYY syndrome had been linked to criminal behaviour in men. Carter expounded:

Again, in the more ordinary field of delinquency and psychopathy, there is the important question of the very early recognition of children at risk, perhaps by the kind of special tests described by Professor Eysenck. These children perhaps shown to be highly introverted and highly neurotic on these same tests should be protected from the additional environmental trauma – such as separation from the mother – that finally pushes them into neurosis or psychosis. (Carter, 1968, pp. 209–10)

This sentiment, that separation from the mother [mothers who don't stay at home where they belong?] causes delinquency is a contemporary version of the preconceptions about motherhood forged at the turn of the century. As usual, the criteria of acceptable motherhood are determined by medical authorities. The agents of the state – the law, the courts, the police in concert with medical professionals and social scientists – decide which women are good mothers and which are not.

The judgement of good motherhood has been predominantly a social judgement of women's social status, sexuality and life-style. Today, the social criteria are expanding with so-called advanced medical knowledge about women's fertility and pregnancy, and about child-rearing. The new genetic technologies create a new definition of genetic 'fitness' and so identify more women as 'needing' genetic technology to breed. The new reproductive technologies result in categorising women as 'egg donors' (genetic mothers), 'carrying mothers' (the women who bears a child), and 'social mothers' (the women who receives a child to rear). Most obviously, the state has taken the opportunity to name women living in a heterosexual union as socially superior mothers. IVF practitioners have been careful to keep within that framework.

Speaking to the Eugenics Society Robert Edwards (1983a) placed the social advantages of IVF in terms of the 'family', mentioning that most couples who undergo IVF are married. He *extended* IVF even further: 'There are some *ethical advantages* in *in vitro* fertilisation' (p. 95 my emphasis). Egg and embryo donation, he said, allow a couple who otherwise have no chance of pregnancy to have their own family. 'The ethical problems may be less because the recipients [sic] must gestate the fetus' (p. 95) Gestating couples?

In the case of a 'surrogate' mother who does not provide the egg, but who receives an IVF 'donor' embryo by embryo transfer, Edwards said, 'The surrogate is transitory, unrelated, a temporary incubator' (p. 96). What happened to physical bonding, physical pregnancy, women's bodies? This is yet another category of motherhood, the surrogate-incubator who losses all status because she has not contributed the 'genetic material' (her own egg) to the pregnancy.

Eugenics and the thinking man

I shall diverge here from reproductive technologies in particular to show how scientists have used theories of heredity and evolution to underpin eugenics.

The English scientist Francis Galton coined the word eugenics in 1883, taking it from the Greek, 'good in stock, hereditarily endowed with noble qualities'. In *Inquiries into the Human Faculty* he explained:

> We greatly want a brief word to express the science of improving stock . . . to give to the more suitable races or strains of blood a better chance of prevailing speedily over the less suitable than they otherwise would have. The word *eugenics* would sufficiently express the idea; it is at least a neater word and a more generalised one than *viriculture,* which I once ventured to use. (Galton, 1883, p. 25)

Viriculture? From the Latin roots, to cultivate the masculine.

Galton and later eugenists were concerned with moral and intellectual faculties (behaviour) not just physical traits. He accepted the influence of environment on human quality (as do today's eugenists), but he concluded from his data the 'vastly preponding effects of nature [inheritance] over nurture'.

Nineteenth-century eugenic principles were synthesised from a complex of interdependent scientific and cultural influences, mainly prevailing theories of evolution and biological theories of inheritance, a cultural concept of 'bloodline descent', changing socio-economic conditions due to industrialisation, and a perceived population problem. In Britain, the belief in 'bloodline' descent affirmed class hierarchy. One's 'blood' identified social standing and determined one's human quality. While the new science of eugenics became the scientific affirmation of the physical and moral superiority of the ruling classes, social radicals simultaneously embraced eugenics to turn the idea of 'blood' inside out. Genetic principles could show the interbreeding among the upper classes as genetically deleterious. Anybody and everybody on the political spectrum could use eugenics to bolster their own interests and social beliefs.

Eugenics became singularly important as a population management strategy. By the ninteenth century the thesis of the political economist Thomas Malthus gained wide acceptance among imperialists in England. In his gloomy essay, *The Principle of Population,* first published anonymously in 1798, Malthus demonstrated mathematically that population was increasing at a faster rate than the means of subsistence. He concluded that population growth was naturally checked by human misery and suffering.[3] His theory aroused population anxiety among the upper classes in England, Europe and North America. In England, one result was a greater policing of the lower classes. For example, the New Poor Laws between 1838 and 1872 forced the most destitute of the population into poor houses, where married women were segregated from their husbands, a kind of no-tech fertility control programme.

Galton addressed the population problem further. He accepted Malthus's thesis, and blamed the overpopulation problem partly on imperialism, 'the filling up of the spare places of the earth which are still void and able to receive the overflow of Europe' (Ibid., p. 318). True to the imperialist mind, he voided the existence of the indigenous populations of non-European cultures. But Galton thought Malthus's assessment was not enough. The problem, he contended, was not only quantity but also the *quality* of the population. This was not a novel idea, as The New Poor Law demonstrates.

Galton talked about 'those whose race we especially want to have' and 'those whose race we especially want to be quit of' (p. 318). He stated outright that in matters of reproduction, religion should relinquish its authority to scientists. He believed this was a matter of importance to the future evolution of the species. Galton was careful to defuse the potential subversive element in eugenic practices: they should not disrupt the prevailing social order. He wrote:

> To sum up in a few words. The chief result of these Inquiries has been to elicit the religious *significance of the doctrine of evolution.* It suggests an alteration in our mental attitude and imposes *a new moral duty.* . . .the new duty which is supposed to be exercised concurrently with, and not in opposition to the old ones upon which the social fabric depends, *is an endeavor to further evolution,* especially that of the human race. (p.337, my emphasis)

The most enthusiastic present-day advocates of reproductive and genetic technologies sustain Galton's beliefs in a scientist-controlled evolution.

In 1961, several of the élite in the scientific community rearticulated Galton's major points in a collection of essays called *The Humanist Frame.*[4] As Galton had, they propounded that there is *a moral duty* for direct human intervention in the course of evolution, and that scientific authority should carry the most weight in this matter. Among the most influential of them were biologist Sir Julian Huxley and the geneticists Conrad H. Waddington and Hermann Muller.

Julian Huxley postulated the new idea system, 'evolutionary humanism'. As he explained, humanism must now be based on scientific knowledge, specifically Darwin's theory of natural selection. Thus, religion was to be displaced by humanism with its secular, rational, scientific, man-centred ethics; and man [his usage] has an ethical responsibility to further the course of evolution (Huxley, 1961a, b).

Waddington (1961) reiterated Huxley's ideas. He compared the all-important evolutionary process of 'natural selection' (favouring the reproduction of certain individuals) with competition between factories in the Industrial Revolution. He added that man's ethical duty was no longer just to control his store of genes, but to invent the type of evolution he wants, and to create novel creatures. Waddington bluntly added that scientists have the knowledge to help in the formulation of a 'supra-ethics', and that human society needs authority [scientists] or else nobody would believe what they were told. Hermann Muller (1961) similarly talked about remoulding organisms in the name of 'progress'. Waddington and Muller placed what would soon be called genetic engineering and reproductive engineering in the scope of Western moral philosophy. They placed their authoritative stamps of approval on reproductive engineering, and they called it a moral imperative, a scientific humanism.

What goes on in women's bodies is the humanist's preserve. Waddington (1961, p. 74) explained 'The biological mechanism of evolution is, as we have said, founded on the genetic transmission of information from parent to offspring through the formation of gametes and their union to form fertilised eggs'. The modern Humanist ethic, whose agenda was set by renowned scientists, created a philosophy which demands the special status of the scientist as ethicist and as engineer of women's reproduction for the sake of human evolution.

Two decades after the publication of *The Humanist Frame*, IVF advocate Clifford Grobstein (1981), US policy commentator and a developmental biologist, echoed the evolutionary 'imperative' in his book *From Chance to Purpose: An Appraisal of External Human Fertilisation*. This book is a philosophical–scientific defence of the use of IVF methods and genetic engineering on women. He calls 'extracorporeal reproduction' (IVF and artificial wombs) the second great step in human evolution (the first step being the acquisition of language). He compares the use of the new reproductive technologies on women with man's quest in outer space. He writes about 'our growing capability to take life into our own hands. That growing capability raises the possibility that some day we shall be able to influence the biological nature of our own species' (p. xi). To engineer the future species of which Grobstein speaks, women's reproduction must be replaced by scientist-controlled reproduction in 'artificial environments', as he calls them. A step forward in the evolutionary humanist ethic.

Grobstein is not considered a raving fanatic. He is a respected 'expert' witness in US government investigations on the NRTs, and he has written for prestigious medical and scientific journals on these issues.

Grobstein's book could be an updated version of *The Humanist Frame*, while *The Humanist Frame* could be an updated version of Galton's *Inquiries into Human Faculty*.

Thus the eugenic uses of artificial reproduction technologies were already set for Edwards and his colleagues by their scientific forebears. Waddington was one of Edwards' mentors. Muller first showed one of the cornerstones of modern genetics, that X-rays cause genetic mutations. Muller also advocated eugenic uses of artificial insemination and IVF. He believed that selective breeding could be accomplished using 'superior' sperm and the insemination of a pool of willing women. He had no doubt that 'enlightened' women would be happy to breed children of great men. He also recognised similar eugenic possibilities in the IVF research of Gregory Pincus in the 1930s. Muller envisaged the fertilisation of 'superior' egg and 'superior' sperm in a laboratory, and the insertion of the embryo into a genetically inferior surrogate mother (Kevles, 1985, p. 189).

Such are the philosophical musings of scientist–eugenists.

The new eugenics. . .depends on genetics

After the Second World War eugenics was reformed.

First, the language of eugenics was depersonalised. The euphemistic term 'genetic counselling' replaced the term 'genetic hygiene' and its negative connotation. Eugenic publications changed their titles. The *Eugenics Quarterly* became the *Journal of Social Biology*. The *Annals of Eugenics* became in 1954 the *Annals of Human Genetics*. Improvement of the 'human stock' was the original aim of eugenics. In the parlance of population genetics, improvement of the human 'gene pool' is the current aim. Instead of talking in terms of race or behavioral traits, eugenists may talk in terms of genetics. Today, we are told, genetic technology of all kinds is beneficial because society bears the burden of 'genetic load' and 'genetic disease' and 'mutational load' and 'genetic risk'. It follows that 'society' must accept genetic intervention, and women should be grateful for the 'medical' technology. Using the gene-oriented language of genetics, doctors and scientists can happily go about their eugenic business disentangled from the past or the questionable present. So, for example, egg 'donation' is considered an acceptable reproductive option for women who are 'carriers' of genetic disease for 'substantially reducing genetic risk' (Carter, 1983b, p. vii).

Second, eugenists made a conscious effort to locate genetic

screening within medicine, where potential parents would find it more acceptable; and coincidentally eugenists promoted placing the subject of genetics in medical school curricula.

Third, with the discovery of the molecular structure of the genetic material DNA in the 1950s came the creation of 'molecular medicine' and 'medical genetics'. (A molecule is a combination of elements or atoms. For a simple example, the molecular formula of water is H_2O. The 'molecules of life', e.g. proteins and DNA, are much larger and more complex.) The incorporation of molecular genetics and molecular biology into medicine changed the face of eugenics. This is the most apparent example of the reorganisation of medicine into a scientific, high-tech, specialised practice. Clinicians are being trained to work side by side with 'basic scientists' who have expertise in gene analysis technology. The molecular revolution in biology masks the symbiotic relationship between eugenics and genetics.

The implications of these three points are conspicuous in the use of genetic screening, which was the first wide-reaching genetic technology to be developed by eugenists with 'selective breeding' applications in mind. The first genetic screening methods were blood tests carried out on potential parents to identify 'carriers' of heritable disease. This capability was followed some years later by pre-natal screening using amniocentesis on pregnant women for detection of fetuses with handicap. By the 1960s, genetic screening was being established in England and the USA. West Germany was slow to implement it because of the negative associations of selective breeding with the Nazi regime (Bradish, 1987), but by the 1970s genetic counselling clinics occurred in many university hospitals there.

We are meant to understand genetic counselling and screening today in terms of its availability as a reproductive choice, at the service of families, mothers, and even for the 'welfare' of the disabled by reducing the numbers who would suffer from a disability. But the motivation behind genetic screening technology was not to offer prospective parents reproductive choice. On the level of social policy, screening was planned for eugenic purposes, to decrease propagation of certain types of people. In the USA, for example, some eugenists suggested that genetic testing of potential parents be made compulsory before marriage, especially for certain racially associated disorders such as Tay Sachs disease, which primarily effects descendents of Central and Eastern European Jews. Perhaps the words of geneticists Luigi Cavalli-Sforza and Walter Bodmer (1971, p. 758) are most revealing: 'In practice, genetic counselling is, to a large extent, really a branch of psychological medicine'.

At about the same time that amniocentesis became available, the abortion laws in Britain and the USA were liberalised, in 1967 and 1973 respectively. Abortion for eugenic reasons, that is if the fetus is judged 'abnormal' by medical tests, was one of the acceptable reasons. The law was adapted to the (doctor-controlled) technology. And the eugenic history of genetic screening has been erased.

Linked to the NRTs, genetic screening technology becomes an even more powerful eugenic tool. For example, at the 1982 Eugenics Society Symposium Cedric Carter suggested a future use of sex-selection of IVF embryos, to screen for female carriers of X-linked genetic disease (see the previous chapter or glossary for an explanation of sex chromosomes and sex-linked disease). Carter (1983c, p. 209) explained the genetic principle that if a man has an X-linked condition such as classical haemophilia, his sons will be unaffected while any daughters he has must be carriers. Thus his daughters are 'at risk of having affected sons and carrier daughters'. Carter infers that in future, when IVF embryos can be identified for sex before insertion in a women's womb, that these female IVF embryos should not be inserted, but rather be discarded, as they pose a 'genetic risk' to the population. His thinking was that the females will grow up and reproduce with their 'faulty' genes, 'risking' producing male children with a genetic condition and female children who are carriers of a genetic condition. Now, this female carrier he is talking about would be perfectly healthy as far as the genetic condition is measured (a 'carrier' does not have the condition, but may pass on a condition to offspring). This is a most presumptuous eugenic tactic, defining us as fit to live according to our reproductive capacity and quality of genes. Eugenic abortion of female carriers is not a novel idea of Carter's. Fourteen years earlier Professor Alan Emery (1968, p. 9) suggested selective abortion of female fetuses detected by amniocentesis for the same situation.

These are examples of 'negative eugenics', the discouragement of 'bad stocks' (as defined by the scholarly Bertrand Russell). There is another sort of eugenics, called positive eugenics, the encouragement of 'good stocks'.

Negative eugenics is not enough for eugenists. The geneticists Luigi Cavalli-Sforza and Walter Bodmer (1971, p. 767) wrote in their textbook *The Genetics of Human Populations*, 'Elimination of genetic defects by negative eugenics is severely limited in its scope. In theory, however, breeding for improvement of desirable traits might give a faster response.' They were talking about artificial insemination of women with selected sperm, what Hermann Muller prescribed as 'germinal choice', and what Julian Huxley called EID, 'Eugenic Insemination by Donor'.

Hermann Muller, among others, proposed the storage of semen of 'excellent men' (sperm banking) for use in a positive eugenics programme. The idea persists today among scientist–eugenists (Beardmore, 1974, p. 114; Carter, 1983c, p. 210).

I learned something interesting reading Cavalli-Sforza and Bodmer's textbook on human genetics. Muller was a Communist for a time, and initially included Lenin and Marx on his list of famous men of 'excellent' genetic endowment. Supposedly, after he became disillusioned with socialism, he removed Lenin and Marx from his list. So much for objectivity. Muller also believed that storing sperm would provide a safeguard against the harmful effects of radiations from nuclear disasters. The 'technical fix' for technical disaster. Today, the same nuclear accident scenario is often included in the arguments for egg and embryo freezing.

As usual, whoever is measuring thinks themselves or those they admire a model of good traits. So, scientists allude to Einstein, Newton, and sometimes Mozart as the kind of people society wants more of. They look forward to reproducing their own kind or, in the case of Mozart, the unthreatening. A Mozart would not challenge scientific authority. The problems with this approach are obvious.

I get the feeling that almost all scientists and medical geneticists who advocate selective breeding think they harbour good genes. 'Intelligence' is the most ubiquitous of 'traits' they are preoccupied with propagating. Of course, they believe they are of the kind 'intelligent', even if they have less praiseworthy hereditary traits, say myopia.

A classic example of the reproducing-the-scientist phenomena is the preponderance of medical students' sperm used for artificial insemination. Apologists (usually medical people) suggest that medical students' sperm is mostly used because they just happen to be around and available and willing. But as the discussion continues, we learn that medical students are considered good sperm donors because they are not off the street, they are considered quite intelligent, and they are knowledgable about their own genetic histories. In other words, any man's sperm wouldn't do. Physicist Robert Graham, the director of the Repository for Germinal Choice in California which stores the sperm of Nobel Laureates and other 'superintelligent' men, reported on a British radio programme, in 1986, that 40 to 50 per cent of the sperm donors are from the medical profession (BBC, 1986). Graham added that he is unable to acquire Black and Asian donors because those he asked did not believe in his programme. Graham's sperm bank is an overextended version of sperm banking generally. Even in a feminist sperm bank in California the donors are screened and typed for an array of abilities, characteristics, and particulars of health and life-style. As Theresia Degener pointed out at the European Women's Conference on Reproductive Technology and Genetic Engineering in Palma, 1986, the Sperm Bank of Northern California may be feminist in its 'open-door' policy to serve all women without discrimination, but it is still eugenic and perpetuates albeism.

The face of eugenics may appear different today than earlier in this century, but the categories remain the same. That is, the 'problem' is still population quality; the aim is still decreasing the number of 'inferior' types, increasing the number of 'desired' types; and the *modus operandi* is still scientific/technological intervention into reproduction.

Discussing the efficacy of eugenics in their textbook on population genetics, Cavalli-Sforza and Bodmer (1971, pp. 753, 757) noted:

> The aim of eugenics is the improvement of the human species by decreasing the propagation of the physically and mentally handicapped (*negative* eugenics) and by increasing that of the 'more desirable' types (*positive* eugenics). It is, in other words, the application to man [sic] of the methods developed by breeders for improving their stocks by artificial selection . . . Some traits such as, for example, inventiveness, artistic talents, and resistance to disease are almost unambiguously favourable and their development should be encouraged, if at all possible. They may, to some extent, be inherited.

These are the same aims and sentiments voiced by eugenists in the past. Even creativity and intellect remain the eugenist–genticist's domain.

There is no doubt that human geneticists in the 1980s see their field and the new genetic technologies in terms of human social 'progress'. On the occasion of receiving a prestigious award in human genetics in 1980 Walter Bodmer (1981, p. 679) said:

Perhaps the revolution that is surely needed in sociology and economics to improve the management of our complex modern society will come from the contributions of biology and biologists to these areas [human genetics]. The whole DNA sequence will eventually be known, and also, but even more eventually, its meaning will be understood. This knowledge will have profound implications for all aspects of human activities and endeavours and surely will, in the long run, contribute positively to the betterment of our society.

Finding the 'DNA sequence' is a controversial scientific project being carried out today (Walsh and Marks, 1986; Palca, 1986; Weatherall, 1985). It entails using genetic engineering methods. The purpose of 'sequencing the human genome' is to elucidate the molecular composition of the entire set of human genes that dwell in the chromosomes. (Taken together, all these genes are called 'the human genome'.)

The above quote from Bodmer's speech was preceded with a reference to his boyhood interest in heredity and people's faces. Bodmer mused, 'Are, therefore, the genes that control facial features *and certain aspects of behaviour* really closely linked to each other' The DNA sequence will no doubt provide the answer in due course' (my emphasis). Whence the revolution in sociology?

Genetic principles are dependent on the values scientists bring to their theorising. Most geneticists agree that environmental and social factors play an important role in human behaviour, and yet they dream on, like Bodmer has, to a genetic theory to explain behaviour and 'drives', and they continue to espouse the application of eugenic–genetic technologies.

Genetics is not neutral. This is nowhere more obvious than in the genetic ideology that permeates the NRTs. For instance, genetic principles have been used to suggest that surrogacy is a genetic phenomenon! In a facile use of evolution theory and sociobiology,[5] the journal *Nature* (1986, p. 95) argued:

> *Procreative instincts* have an adaptive significance for all species and . . . cannot be repressed by legislation [prohibiting surrogacy]. Moreover, it is *natural* that couples should prefer genetically related to unrelated children: Dawkin's concept of the selfish gene, not to mention a great deal of sociobiology, refers . . . (It seems to be common ground that the willingness of some women to bear children for close relatives, another illustration of the selfishness of genes, should not be prevented by law if no money changes hands.) (My emphasis)

To explain, ethologist Richard Dawkins wrote in *The Selfish Gene* (1978), 'We are survival machines – robot vehicles blindly programmed to preserve the selfish molecules known as genes. This is a truth . . .' (p. x).

The concept of the 'selfish gene' is controversial even among scientists, but *Nature* portrays it as an accepted scientific fact. Worse, the scientific assessment portrays women as genetically driven to reproduce. It obscures cultural reality, the social relations affecting women's relationship to pregnancy, birth, and childrearing. The desire for offspring is a malleable human quality, a part of human society and culture, not a genetically determined one. Mothers of adopted children refer.

Christine Crowe (1987a) has spoken to women on IVF programmes. Many of them related that they would have been happy to adopt, but their male partners were unwilling. The men preferred their own genetic offspring, even when the other 'option' meant that the women would have to undergo IVF treatment and all it entails. In these cases, the 'genetic drive' explanation imposes a male reality; it buttresses the importance of biological paternity.

The selfish gene assessment from a credible scientific journal, and one whose editorial policy has power in the establishment of policy,[6] is shocking, yet typical of their utter disregard for 'non-scientific' experience (what women do) and their high regard for scientific concepts gleaned from scientific theory-making and experimentation. Their use of a genetic theory deflates the science-is-neutral palliative, as one academic put it, 'We should consider the genetic hypothesis calmly and dispassionately, for in itself it has no practical political consequence whatsoever' (Durant, 1984).

Population and depopulation

The political importance of global population control projects cannot be overstressed. The perceived global 'population problem' is a eugenic anxiety.

The birth control movement and development of contraceptive technology was caught up in the eugenics movement.[7] Contraceptive pill pioneer Gregory Pincus was finally convinced to pursue research on a hormonal contraceptive out of recognition of the 'overpopulation' problem, not women's 'right to choose' (see Pincus, 1965). Family planning, as birth control became known, gained acceptance from scientists, doctors, and politicians when its population control possibilities were appreciated, that is when it was clear that it could be used to control women's fertility. As they saw it, contraception technology could check the overpopulation problem in general, and the 'overbreeding' of the poor in particular.

In *The Genetics of Human Populations* Cavalli-Sforza and Bodmer (1971) stated the links between one kind of population control (quantity control) and another kind (quality control). From their scientific perspective they wrote that because of the 'population explosion', 'man is confronted today with another motive for controlling his reproduction'. They stressed the need to generate the 'right attitude' towards birth control among the entire human species. 'If we can learn how to do this we may in the process also learn to introduce eugenic considerations, for similar human attitudes are required for both' (p. 757). They name genetic counselling as 'another kind of reason for limiting human reproduction'. In short, a modern eugenics is justified in the 1970s for them because of the 'population explosion' and because genetic screening exists.

What they do not make clear is that population control technology is applied differently towards the women of Western and 'Third World' countries, and that in industralised countries such as the USA and Britain, different groups of women have had different experiences of birth control. What they do not make clear is that their population control ideals subordinate women to eugenic aims.

Racist and eugenic practices underpinning the birth control movement have been documented (for examples see Gordon, 1976; and Kevles, 1985). Linda Gordon, in *Women's Body, Women's Right: A Social History of Birth Control in America* (1976) discussed the racism in certain birth control clinics in the early days of the movement, and examples of 'an apartheid system of birth control: different devices prescribed for whites and blacks' (p. 309). The fuel for this kind of treatment was the contention by some of the most ardent birth control pioneers that Black women were of lower intelligence than White women.

At the Emergency Conference on the New Reproductive Technologies in 1985, Sultana Kamal spoke of the interrelationships between the use of the new technology of IVF in the West and the use of contraceptive technology on 'Third World' women:

> With the origination and projected expansion of the new reproductive technologies in the West along with the obsessive emphasis on population control in the Third World countries, the international as well as the national population policies need to be examined in a new light . . . It is also essential to see . . . how both are linked through principles of selective breeding to entice 'the fit' to breed and to restrain reproduction by 'the unfit'. To me, the promotion of technologies having exactly opposite purposes in different parts of the world is in fact aimed at a common goal, that is control over human reproductive power. (Kamal, 1987, p. 146)

Both Sultana Kamal and Farida Akhter stress that the introduction of Western birth control technology in foreign aid packages is not liberating to the women of their country, Bangladesh. Contraceptive technologies and population control programmes do not allow women there to make decisions about their lives and their reproduction. Destitute women are being coerced to accept sterilisation in exchange for food, or to accept dangerous experimental long-term hormonal contraceptives as the only 'choices'. Hormonal contraceptives and IUDs are administered without health examinations or follow-up care. The aid agency USAid which supports many development programmes in Bangladesh advised the government not to attach the population control programme to health care administration as it would slow down family planning 'progress'. Menstrual regulation, a form of birth control acceptable to some women in Bangladesh, has been banned in many areas because the Reagan-headed US government is not willing to grant aid money for abortion-like methods (see Akhter, 1987, 1986a, 1986b; and Kamal, 1987).

In Farida Akhter's words, the purpose of the Western-controlled population strategies in developing countries is not a population policy but a *depopulation* policy. Western population anxiety over the birth rate in developing countries reflects Western cultural, ideological, and technological imperialism. It is a differential interpretation of Malthus: people in the West have a divine 'right' to multiply and consume; the rest of the world succumbs to the miserable fate of Malthus' prediction and must be 'saved' from overreproducing and from messing up the world for privileged consumers in the West. The problems in former colonial territories are not due to 'overpopulation', they are due to racism and overexploitation. Akhter relates how once fertile fields in Bangladesh now lie in waste because of colonial exploitation, while today shrimps are caught for export to European countries while the poorest people of Bangladesh starve.

The fundamental issue for women, of course, is that all over the world we would like to control our own sexuality and reproduction. We would like to decide when to have children, to space pregnancies, not to become pregnant unexpectedly. The problem is not, as it seems from the male view in all this, birth control technology or no birth control technology. The problem is patriarchy, the social conditions which place women in economic and social dependence on husbands, fathers, religion, the state and its male dominated institutions including medical science. In the global politics of population control, it is patriarchal social relations in its various guises which are standing in the way of women's control of our own reproductive capacities.[8]

A few examples from the 1973 Eugenics Society Symposium *Population and the New Biology* illustratrate the nature of international eugenic population control. I use these examples in particular because they are given among papers on IVF, AID, and genetic screening, clearly illustrating how all the technologies of reproduction play distinctive roles in maintaining national and international interests.

British civil servant C. M. Stewart (1974, p. 114), speaking on the 'population problem' in Britain, noted that 'within the next generation some formal consideration of population quality, as well as quantity, will need to form part of any government policy on population'. This includes, we later find out, 'measures to discourage the reproduction of at least some of the patently handicapped'. Consider this statement in light of the claim that pre-natal screening is an optional, free choice.

In *The Future of Oral Contraception* (1974) biologist Clive Wood repeated the kind of judgements we have come to expect from mainstream policy commentators: hormonal contraceptives are appropriate for use on women in 'Third World' countries because of the shortage of health care workers. It frees the paramedics time! His thinking endorses another 'technical fix', where women pay with their health and autonomy for a social resourse problem. Concerning women in the West, the author acknowledged 'unpleasant' side effects of a DES (diethylstilbestrol) contraceptive, but he cites studies showing that the risks of pregnancy outweigh the risks of the Pill. The comparison is like comparing apples and oranges. Why is the choice measured between the risks of pregnancy and the risks of hormonal contraceptives, as if those are comparable and the only alternatives? As for the 'unpleasant' effects of the synthetic estrogen drug DES, these include an increased risk of breast cancer in women who take it, which may not develop until twenty years later. Also, if traces of DES linger in a woman's body when she is pregnant, there is the risk of reproductive tract abnormalities in her daughters and sons, including a rare form of vaginal cancer in daughters (Direcks, 1987).

Mass voluntary sterilisation was discussed in another paper as an answer to the overconsumption problem in the USA (Free and Duncan, 1974, p. 65). No one proposed that an answer to overconsumption is less consumption. While for the 'Third World', the authors consider sterilisation better than trying to follow up repetitive contraceptive procedures. This is not about women's welfare, women's control of our reproductive capacities or social justice. Although the authors recognise the effect of social factors, malnutrition and discrimination, *the recognition merely fuels the arguments for technological manipulation of reproduction.* Any 'sensitivity' and 'compassion' these commentators avow is shallow, existing within the framework of racism and sexism, and depends on keeping developing countries in a dependent place, and women everywhere at the service of eugenists.

In summary, the NRTs follow in eugenic footsteps, compromising women's integrity, rights, and freedom. At the turn of the century population engineering was deemed crucial to Empire. Today, population engineering is deemed necessary in Western countries to 'maintian' the human species in the framework of White male cultural supremacy.[9]

In 1892, Francis Galton wrote of the eugenics movement, 'We may not be able to originate, but we can guide' (p. xxvii). Less than a hundred years later scientists are aiming to *originate* genetic 'improvement' with reproductive and genetic engineering technologies. IVF, cloning, sex determination are 'the creation of life by new means' and the new technologies 'could enable the formation of many individuals with a desired genotype [genetic make-up]' (Hemsworth, 1974, pp. 5, 15). The scientist-creator takes centre stage.

8

A matter of state interest

Reproductive and genetic technologies are a matter of state interest. The new reproductive technologies (NRTs) are powerful tools of 'human reproduction' and so for social intervention in families and population control, the modern eternal preoccupation of nations.

The new biotechnologies can, however, disrupt the social order and existing ideologies of the family. Removing women's eggs from our bodies and fertilising them in a laboratory, and perhaps inserting them into another confused old definitions of motherhood. With the expansion of *in vitro* fertilisation (IVF) methods, with more stages of pregnancy taking place outside the woman's body and in a laboratory, women's role in reproduction is being altered. What will happen to the image of motherhood, the bulwark of sexism on which the state depends to deny female citizens full humanity and citizenship in the name of 'embryos' and the 'family'? Given the potential social problems, the state is interested in resolving the tension between the ideology of the family and the technology of reproduction. As we will see, governments understand that the NRTs can serve to reassert the 'normality' of patriarchal social relations, and are willing to accept NRTs for precisely this reason.

The complexities and powers of high technology – any technology – demand organisation and regulation of some kind. The existence of the NRTs have provided governments with another reason to interfere with human reproduction in the guise of protection.

For medical scientists and the state the question of control is, how much power will the state retain in the implementation of reproductive technology, and how much power will science and medicine retain? It is not a fundamental difference of opinion over the use of women or the eugenic uses of the NRTs. On those two issues the scientific establishment and the state are in agreement.

Governments purport to be involved in regulating reproductive technology in the interests of 'society', reflecting in democratic societies the wishes of the 'public'. That public is not women. Institutions such as the church, the social services and law societies are granted a role by governments in defining the acceptable level of scientific intervention in reproduction. Women as a class do not share power in that sphere.

By the state I mean the government and the agents of the state, that is the institutions involved in organising and regulating society. The state asserts itself through legislation, legitimation of power, formal and informal sanctions. Science is an institution today, more powerful and organised than ever before. The state empowers science, while science serves state interests, as for example in the fields of atomic physics, information technology, chemical and biological warfare and contraception technologies. In turn, scientists receive positions of authority in society, political posts, and a large measure of authority over themselves with respect to research projects and development of technologies.

The overlapping fraternal interests and collaboration of the state and medical science are important points here. Although the interests of medical science and governments are distinct, their fraternal interests are similar. The technologies embody male-stream values; they are a means of maintaining class and gender hierarchies; they require the subordination of women. This is part of the explanation for the fact that today dissimilar governments, right, left and centre politically, whether capitalist or socialist, are coming to similar assessments about the meaning and use of reproductive technologies.

By the early 1980s, the intense controversy and confusion surrounding the whole IVF area prompted many governments to establish official inquiries into IVF issues, including egg and embryo donation, freezing of eggs and embryos, artificial insemination (AI), surrogacy, human embryo research, the use of genetic engineering in women's reproduction. These committees were charged with investigating and analysing the new advances in reproductive technology and making recommendations so that governments could then act on them knowledgeably. An aim of these committees was to allay 'public anxiety', as the British Warnock Committee stated. Or as Norwegian lawyer Anne Hellum interprets, they act as public tranquilisers.[1]

Governments have signalled their acceptance of the new reproductive and genetic technologies in the reports of official government inquiries. These reports reflect the views of agents of the state, such as medical scientists, lawyers, and professional ethicists and social scientists. The reports are not mere bureaucratic stamps of approval or disapproval of new methods. They are pivotal in the formation of policy towards reproductive practice, defining the role and power of medicine and science over women, and most fundamentally in approving the meaning of scientific reproduction.

To examine government intent in the reproductive technology area, in this chapter I look at some of these government committees, some of their legal aspects, and what they mean for women. I will explore their meaning of 'medical therapy' and regulation of reproductive and genetic technologies.

Government inquiries have been established world-wide on various levels: on the provincial level in Australia and Canada; on the national level in Britain, West Germany, Denmark, Sweden, Spain and several other countries; on an international level in the European Parliament. In the USA the only federal government report on *in vitro* fertilisation was issued in 1979 by the Ethics Advisory Board of the Department of Health, Education and Welfare (now the Department of Health and Human Services). The Ethics Advisory Board disbanded in 1980 creating a *de facto* ban on government funding of IVF research in the USA. Since then USA Congressional hearings have been held on gene therapy and on *in vitro* fertilisation and embryo freezing. I do not refer directly to these hearings in this chapter, instead I cite a US non-government ethics report which mimics the government reports in other countries. It is the report of the American Fertility Society – a medical society.

I concentrate on English language reports, especially on the British Committee of Inquiry into Human Embryology and Reproduction in Britain. The report of that committee, called the Warnock Report, has been most influential in Britain and in other countries. Professional medical and scientific bodies have taken it as a point of reference and other governments named the Warnock

Committee as a model for their own committees. All the government reports published as of 1987 take a similar approach to the NRTs. They all endorse the use of IVF on women as medical therapy and research on human embryos, including genetic research.

Structure and function of the government committees

The structure of the committees reflects the empowering of various kinds of 'experts' to define the boundaries of reproductive technology. Several government committees established in the mid-1980s were multidisciplinary panels of professionals. Two of these were the British Warnock Committee and the Victoria (Australia) Waller Committee. By contrast, the Ontario (Canada) investigation was carried out by the Ontario Law Reform Commission comprised of five male lawyers. However, they in turn appointed a multidisciplinary Advisory Board to assist them.

The relationship between the government commissioners and medical scientists in this matter is intimate. The technologies themselves are to a large extent defined by scientific 'experts', the same professionals whose interests are served by allowing the practice of IVF and human embryo research. Medical scientists act as members of inquiries and as 'expert' witnesses to them. In turn, it is in the interest of IVF doctors and scientists to share authority with governments in the area of women's reproduction. By taking an early and aggressive role in the formulation of government policy, scientists have influenced the limitations and mode of regulation.

The chair of the British Warnock Committee was moral philosopher Dame Mary Warnock, now Baroness Warnock. The remaining fifteen members of the committee included professionals in law, medicine, natural science, social science, theology and ethics. The members included Anne McLaren, an embryologist who conducts *in vitro* research on animals and is Director of the Medical Research Council Mammalian Development Unit; David Davies a former editor of *Nature*, which serves as a mouthpiece for the scientific establishment; and Professor of Obstetrics and Gynaecology Sir Malcolm C Macnaughton, who has carried out research on human fetuses *in vitro* (acquired from late-term abortions), is the director of the IVF centre at the Royal Infirmary in Glasgow, and has been President of the RCOG since 1984. Scientific interests were well represented on the committee. Women with fertility problems, women who 'carry' genetic disease, women who might be potential egg donors, women who might be surrogate mothers, and representatives of women's groups were not members of the committee.

Since the public is invited to submit evidence, committees of inquiry in Great Britain should provide a mechanism for public participation in government. However, no women's group in Britain was *invited* to give oral evidence on issues concerning fertility, pregnancy and motherhood. Instead the committee invited such evidence from organisations and institutions, like the Royal College of Obstetricians and Gynaecologists (RCOG), to speak authoritatively about women's concerns. The RCOG is no friend of women. For example, they have acted to restrict and control women's access to abortion, identifying themselves as moral arbiters and experts in this regard (see RCOG *et al.*, 1985 and Chapter 4).

The so-called science 'experts' are preoccupied with protecting their own interests, not women's. In Britain, their recurring question has been, how will regulation of IVF and genetic technology affect scientific freedom? The reaction of scientists to the statutory regulations on 'human embryo research' (experiments on women) illustrates this point. IVF pioneers Robert Edwards and Patrick Steptoe, and two major scientific bodies, the Medical Research Council (MRC) and the Royal Society, argued against a fourteen-day upper limit for human embryo research. Edwards and Steptoe suggested a longer time limit, the MRC suggested a different way of defining a limit, and the Royal Society wanted a more flexible [open ended] limit. Further, the research science establishment, including the ever editoralising journal *Nature*, decried statutory regulation of the fourteen-day limit, as the Warnock Committee proposed.

The science 'experts' identify themselves as the agents of the state, regulators rather than representatives of the women on whom these techniques are used. An editorial in *Nature* (1984) stated that the Warnock Committee recommendations for regulation of AID (artificial insemination by donor) are 'less stringent than they might be', because genetic data about donors should be available to researchers. Their message is: less government regulation of embryo researchers in the intersts of scientists, but more regulation of AID, again in the interests of scientists.

The Warnock Committee recommended regulation of the NRTs, including AID, through a centralised 'licensing and storage authority' which must include a substantial membership of non-scientists. They added that any non-licensed activity should be a criminal offence. In 1985, the MRC and the RCOG established the Voluntary Licensing Authority (VLA) along the lines the Warnock Report recommended, while they awaited government action on Warnock recommendations. The MRC and RCOG jointly nominated the several lay (non-medical/non-scientist) members. So, medical science is being regulated by medical scientists. This has been the case all along. Guidelines for IVF and human embryo research initially come from medical science sources.

Reminiscing about the 1970s ethical debates over IVF, Robert Edwards (1980d, pp. 115–16) commented:

I would not wish the reader to imagine we [Edwards and Steptoe] were over-vulnerable. I had been a member of a small committee for some years now that had been formed to *clarify ethical issues* arising from advances in biology. Its Chairman was Walter Bodmer, *Professor of Genetics at Oxford University*. It included a theologian, Gordon Dunstan, John Maddox, who was *editor of* Nature . . . *Doctors and scientists like myself* held numerous meetings and we called on many witnesses to discuss organ transplantation, the screening of fetuses for inherited disorders, artificial insemination and, of course, fertilisation *in vitro*. (My emphasis).

In previous chapters we met up with Edwards and Steptoe and population geneticist Walter Bodmer, a principle promoter of the social and eugenic usefulness of the NRTs. Bodmer was also appointed to the working party of the Council for Science and Society to investigate IVF issues. Their report, published shortly before the Warnock Report in 1984, favoured 'human embryo' experimentation for up to six weeks after fertilisation; the report also considered some kinds of surrogacy arrangements justifiable. John Maddox does not appear by name in this book, but he was editor of *Nature* at the time of their editorial campaign promoting the NRTs in the 1980s, and so is accountable for the content of those editorials which I have been quoting. The Rev Gordon Dunstan, an admirer of Robert Edwards, presented a paper on the NRTs at the Eugenics Society Symposium in London, in 1982, when Edwards gave the keynote Galton Lecture. Dunston also chaired the Council for Science and Society working party reviewing IVF issues. He subsequently became a member of the Voluntary Licensing Authority set up to oversee IVF practice and research. As you can see, in many cases the same advocates of the NRTs regularly appear on the most important 'expert' committees investigating the issues.

The centralised licensing authority recommended by the Warnock Committee will oversee the experts to their own tune. Equally important it guarantees that a small number of scientists and their hand-picked lay members control the technologies. If the Warnock recommendations become law, it means women's self-help groups and the role of unlicensed doctors (non-specialists) will be severely restricted. The VLA agrees that any unlicensed practice should be made a criminal offence. The policy decisions being made in reproductive technology reflect the ever growing entitlement of scientists to participate in the formulation and implementation of state intervention in the family and society. Ignoring women and recognising science allowed the Warnock Committee to place control of technologies in the hands of medical scientists once acceptable boundaries are set *with major input by medical scientists and their apologists sitting on the government committee in the first place.*

Fertility problems and embryos

Early on in their reports, government committees state their judgement that infertility is a malfunction, a disease, an illness, a tragedy. This is a crucial judgement, since it opens the door to their other considerations. The Warnock Committee judged that infertility is a 'malfunction' of couples (p. 9). From that, they judged that artificial reproduction technologies, AID and certain IVF methods, are appropriate *medical* treatment. They reserve the use of reproductive and genetic technologies as 'medical therapy'. Thus they expand further the definition and jurisdiction of the practice of medicine. From there, they agreed with IVF experts that the aims of

IVF treatment also include the reduction of congenital and hereditary disorders, and the development of contraceptive methods. The Ontario Law Reform Commission (1985) admitted that IVF is not the practice of medicine, since IVF methods are performed by scientists who are not doctors. They approved an 'expanding and flexible' concept of medicine (p. 34ff).

The Warnock Committee did not address the complex medical and psychosocial aspects of infertility, the cultural aspects that certainly affect women and men, the causes and medical treatments. Instead, the committee followed the path of the IVF 'experts' preoccupied with the prestigious technology.

The Warnock Committee approved the use of IVF for infertility treatment, but only for heterosexual couples living together in stable relationships. Their reason for denying the services to lesbians and single women was simply, 'We believe that as a general rule it is better for children to be born into a two-parent family, with both father and mother' (p. 11). Their message is, women are subversive when not adhering to traditional definitions of motherhood and sexuality. They approve one kind of family and sexuality over others for *moral* reasons. Most other countries also limit availability of IVF to married couples, or couples living in a marriage type relationship, 'in the best interests of the child', although the Ontario Law Reform Commission stated that they are sensitive to discrimination against single women and so lists 'stable single women' among those who should be eligible (p. 45). However, this eligibility is tentative. They added that the final authority on who is 'stable' (fit to breed) lies with the courts and the medical profession, and that it is appropriate for the courts to consider marital status in making their judgements.

The policy debate on the NRTs gives the state the opportunity to name the 'family' (that is one kind of family, heterosexual couples) as better than women ourselves in 'the best interests of the child', and then to ban or control any activities which challenge that. The assessment is dangerous for women. Not only does it discriminate against certain women, but most significantly it defines 'fitness' for all women, not only for women on IVF programmes. It challenges the mothering of any woman not living with a man by setting up a morally superior womanhood, that is attached to men.

The Warnock Report repeatedly infers specific definitions of good womanhood. The report leaves the impression that a moral couple is one who would use the NRTs to avoid abortion. It argues that IVF offers a better approach than abortion in cases of known genetic 'risk' to offspring, giving the example that a woman who is a 'carrier' of genetic disease could enter an IVF programme and receive donor eggs from another woman, and so bypass the problem of choosing an abortion. (To explain, abortion is allowed, and often encouraged, for negative eugenic reasons, that is if the fetus is shown to be 'abnormal' by pre-natal screening). These technologies are not only about managing infertility for heterosexual couples, they are about avoiding abortion as well. Women are not recognised as being capable of making moral decisions about abortion (about ourselves) on our own authority. The embryo needs protection from women. The medical profession acts as the agent of the state in providing that protection by controlling abortion on two fronts; a woman must receive permission from two doctors to be allowed an abortion in Britain, and now, medical scientists can control the conditions of women's reproduction through IVF and have women bypass abortion. Meanwhile, medical scientists are allowed to discard IVF embryos or handle them experimentally for a time. IVF practitioners are allowed under their own authority to cause numerous 'extra-uterine' abortions, if you will.

The pro-technology minded majority on the committee ignored the moral paradox of allowing scientists to handle embryos and inevitably discard many of them, while the criminalisation of abortion denies pregnant women reproductive self-determination in the name of embryo protection. The committee never acknowledged that the issues could be linked to the abortion debate. Rather, they took the attitude of IVF 'experts' playing into the hands of anti-abortionists, that human embryo research and IVF are the antithesis of abortion, the creation of life. The rhetoric of these reports revolves around embryos, scientific knowledge, and a certain view of good womanhood.

The Swedish government report *Genetisk Integritet* (Genetic Integrity) does mention the abortion connection, concluding that in the case of abortion the value of the embryo is inferior to a woman's right to self-determination with regard to her body. They still, however, create a separate identity for embryos. This leaves room for their considerations on embryo interests and the use of genetic technology on embryos.

In the name of the 'family'

Disregard for women's integrity, health and well-being, can be seen in the way the various government committees assessed IVF, egg donation, surrogacy, and human embryo research. In the Warnock Report, approval or disapproval of particular techniques had little to do with the medical risk involved and more to do with whether the technique was considered socially useful or not. This is apparent in their inconsistent evaluation of risk factors associated with a particular IVF procedure.

The Warnock Committee considered IVF for heterosexual couples mostly unproblematic ethically. Physical risks to women undergoing IVF (invasive hormonal treatment, anaesthesia, laparoscopy for surgical removal of eggs, ultrasound, amniocentesis, and probably Caesarean section) were dismissed as minor risks in a preliminary discussion of the IVF procedure. Their judgement that IVF is in this case ethical was caught up in their thinking that infertility is a malfunction that requires medical treatment. They never addressed the fact that IVF is used for subfertility in men. In such cases, a perfectly healthy fertile woman by medical standards is being given IVF with little mention of the risk to her, perhaps even risk of becoming infertile herself from the IVF procedure. It is not an unlikely possibility that the IVF procedure might cause reproductive system problems in the woman undergoing treatment, considering that IVF entails biochemical and mechanical manipulation of the woman's reproductive organs.

The physical risks of IVF are finally mentioned as an argument against egg donation by surgical retrieval of eggs. Thus, on the one hand, the Warnock Committee consider that the risks of IVF are minor for the infertile woman, or fertile woman whose male partner has fertility problems. On the other hand, they recognise the risks of the procedure with respect to an 'egg donor' woman. It is most significant that their consideration of the risk to women of IVF depends on a woman's status with respect to a man. The risk is not recognised in the same way in the case of a woman in a relationship with a man (remember the Warnock Committee from the start of their discussion is only considering IVF procedures for women living with men in marital-type relationships).

Still, despite the risks to the 'egg donor' woman, the Committee approved egg donation by surgical retrieval of eggs anyway because of its overall *social* value. They stated that egg donation is beneficial because (i) it provides an offspring which is genetically related to the husband, and (ii) women who carry heritable genetic disease can bypass using their own eggs and use another woman's eggs instead. Egg donation allows a semblance of a 'natural' (genetic) family and it can be used to control the types of children born.

The eugenic–genetic point is important. The Warnock Committee did not question their policy of negative eugenics, the burdens it places on women and couples, nor its implications for the disabled. Having accepted the importance of 'genetic health', egg donation by surgery is a 'logical' and 'acceptable' eugenic tool for them. Let me stress that the Warnock Committee projects itself as having carried out a rigorous, scholarly investigation of IVF issues. The committee members were high-powered professionals who should have been aware of various studies and criticisms on the issue of 'genetic health' coming from the women's health movement and the disability rights movement, as well as individuals.

In Australia, the Victoria Waller Committee warned that women who are potential egg donors (women undergoing gynaecological or abdominal surgery) may be reluctant to disappoint doctors. But in the end both they and the Ontario Law Reform Commission approved the use of IVF and egg donation on the basis of an individual's 'right-to-treatment' and the often used logic that egg donation is the same as sperm donation.

Having accepted egg donation by surgical removal of eggs, the Warnock Committee rejected egg donation by uterine lavage, by which a woman conceives in her body usually by artificial insemination with sperm from the husband/male partner of the receiving couple. If all goes as planned, the fertilised egg is 'washed out' of the woman's womb and inserted into the womb of the receiving woman. The Warnock Committee cites physical risks to the 'donor' woman as the reason they reject lavage. But considering their expedient use of 'risk' in the context of IVF methods, the evident reason uterine lavage is rejected is the problem of an unplanned pregnancy if the fertilised egg implants in the woman's uterine wall. What can society do with this woman? The confusion of relationships challenges the exclusivity of marriage. If she has an abortion she is not a 'good' woman; if she carries the child and keeps it, then the father of her offspring is somebody else's husband; and if she carries the child and gives it up to the couple, she is acting as a 'surrogate' mother, which is not acceptable to the Warnock Committee. There is no respectable place in Britain for this woman in the usual categories of motherhood.

A pattern emerges. IVF technologies can stabilise the social order by helping to maintain nuclear family units. The NRTs can serve to reaffirm the 'normality' of the patriarchal family.

The explicit genetic argument, that it is better to have your own genetic offspring, is used by government committees over and over again to approve the use of IVF, egg donation, sperm donation in IVF, embryo donation, and 'surrogacy'.

Just as IVF practitioners have argued, so have the Warnock, Waller and Ontario Committees suggested that IVF technology solves the shortcomings of adoption. Reasons they give for the use of IVF and gamete or embryo donation are that (i) adoption is no longer an available option for childless couples due to the shortage of babies; (ii) having one's own genetic child or one that is matched for characteristics to the parents is more desirable than adoption; and (iii) as the Ontario Law Reform Commission bluntly states, regular adoption is socially intrusive to families (Warnock Report, 1984, pp. 9, 40; Waller Report (b), 1983, p. 14; Ontario Law Reform Commission, 1985, pp. 14, 28). The message is, women's bodies may be biochemically and physiologically manipulated to overcome the social 'problems' of adoption.

Thus, the new reproductive technologies are logical in a world where women are related to men and the 'family', not to ourselves as women. The NRTs fabricate an essential coupledom. Heterosexual couples living together, socially and economically interdependent, are so essential *at this time in history* to reproductive technologies that the word 'couple' appears in a list of definitions in the American Fertility Society report, *Ethical Considerations of the New Reproductive Technologies* (1986). The Warnock Report uses the words husband and wife to mean the individuals in the couple, whether married or not. From there, *women's risks, rights, interests, role, authority (non-authority) is defined in relation to coupledom.* Legal considerations – and legal status – follow suit. This viewpoint undermines women's identity as autonomous persons, and again defines women as wives and mothers in legal and moral dependence on men.

Paternity anxiety

One intention of the regulators of the new reproductive technologies is of social/scientific control of reproduction. This is apparent in the way that AID and surrogacy are handled similarly to IVF and genetic engineering. Both AID and surrogacy, essentially non-'technical' methods of reproduction, are being redefined in government reports as 'technology' which warrants medical science 'expert' control.

'Artificial insemination' has been around for at least a few hundred years, and possibly longer. Insemination requires no technical expertise and no scientific knowledge. Any woman with access to sperm can carry it out without the assistance of the medical profession, and many women do use insemination as a reproductive option. It is referred to as 'self-insemination' or simply 'insemination' and can be done at home. Women can do it alone, and unregulated insemination offers women a measure of control over reproduction.

The way in which AID is being assessed and regulated is an obvious example of government intent to further control women's reproduction in the service of patriarchal social relations. The Warnock Committee, and every other government committee on the subject of IVF, have included artificial insemination in the realm of reproductive technology. By including insemination with IVF they could redefine a controversial social practice into a high-tech medical procedure. The Warnock Report stated the problem outright: artificial insemination was included in an inquiry prompted by 'test-tube' baby methods because it 'is not universally accepted ethically, nor indeed regulated by law' (p. 5).

The Warnock Committee proposed that AI be regulated for moral reasons by the same central licensing authority required to regulate IVF, a complex procedure that entails sophisticated technical skill, physical risks for the woman receiving treatment, and unique ethical implications. Regulating AID in Britain along the lines the Warnock Report recommends would mean that only cohabiting heterosexual women would have access to AID sevices and only for medically defined reasons. It would mean that women who organise self-insemination groups in England would be criminally liable. Physicians would require a special licence to offer AID. And research scientists could have access to donated sperm for their genetic studies, just as they have access to gametes (eggs and sperm) from IVF programmes. Regulated AID gives the state and medical science greater control over women's reproduction, but it gives women less control.

The Ontario Law Reform Commission obtained the same effect by categorising AI with IVF as 'non-conventional therapy', where by 'conventional therapy' they meant anything from infertility counselling to highly invasive hormonal treatment and surgical interventions. Calling AI 'non-conventional', then, has nothing to do with the sophisitication of the medical intervention, but depends on a social appraisal of AID and IVF as 'artificial' (non-coital). The commission stated that AI must be regulated to 'preclude unqualified persons from undertaking the procedure' (p. 30). To substantiate the medicalisation of AI they claimed associated medical risks: penetration of the cervix, complications from the possible injection of air, 'severe reactions' [none are given], and possible death. These claims are ridiculous in the context in which presented.

AID concerns overlap IVF concerns for the state, not because it is a technological intervention into reproduction *per se*, but because (i) any woman's behaviour which challenges the concept of the natural patriarchal order is a concern of the state, (ii) any woman's reproductive behaviour which is beyond the control of men destabilises medical and state authority over women, and (iii) AID can be used as a eugenic, quality control tool of medical scientists, for example by screening of sperm donors for genetic 'information'.

The cheat is that neither medical science nor government committees acknowledge some women's experiences of using AI, experience as single mothers, experience as lesbian mothers, or the lives of their children. Instead, we get the story from government commissioners that it is 'not in the best interests of children' (read: there is no identifiable father with rights), and equally ludicrous, that it is a specialist medical procedure and must be regulated as such.

Moves to regulate AID are caught up in the state's preoccupation with paternity and identifying a father. The Warnock Report recommends changing the law so that the husband of the woman receiving AID would be the legal father of the offspring. The change in the law would change the status of the resulting child from illegitimate to legitimate. The question of paternity has been the biggest obstacle in the social and legal approval of AID as 'non-coital reproduction'. This is not a new development. The laws in many countries have been or are being 'reformed' to name the consenting social father as the legal father when a woman becomes pregnant by AID.

Legitimising the AID child (not all children) is the codification in law yet again of the rights and privileges of the father, and the meaning of patrilineal inheritance. Only fathers can legitimise. The concept of illegitimacy regulates women's sexual and social behaviour and dependency on men. It legitimises patriarchal family relations, the idea of children as a male property right. It arises from the ultimate disregard for women. Under an old English common law, the child of a woman without a husband was considered *filius nullius*, 'no one's child'.

One reason lawyers have been recommending changing the laws regarding legitimacy with respect to AID is that some women who give birth to children conceived by AID have been naming their husbands or male partners as the legitimate fathers on birth certificates anyway. The state, as the keeper of significant 'biological facts' like births, deaths, marriages (paternity), is not in control if women and couples choose to flaunt the biological 'facts'. Another reason for changing the law is to counter the growing numbers of women unattached to men who use insemination as a reproductive option. In Sweden the law now states that a woman seeking AID services must have the written consent of a man.

Not one of the government committees on the NRTs takes the opportunity to recommend the most decent answer of all, that the sexist, classist notion of illegitimacy be discarded altogether.[2]

The question of paternal authority is inevitably posed again in the context of IVF. A pointed example of the preoccupation with paternal inheritance was the Warnock Committee's recommendations about the location of an embryo in the event of the death of the father. As they stated, the AIH (artificial insemination with husband's sperm) or IVF child not *in utero* at the date of the father's death should be 'disregarded for purposes of succession to and inheritance from the [father]' (p. 55). Anticipating unprecedented legal complications resulting from the use of frozen embryos they added, 'for the purposes of establishing primogeniture the date and time of birth, and not the date of fertilisation, shall be the determining factor' (p. 57). The message from the Warnock

Committee is that the male-headed social order will be protected against the disruptive effect of artificial reproduction techniques. Statutory measures on the status of children conceived by artificial reproduction technologies not only protect the interests of the individual males involved, they solidify the interests of all males in the society

For example, in the case of AID, when it is better *not* to define the genetic father as the legal father, the law will oblige the social father. But this assessment does not negate the rights of the genetic father over mothers in other contexts. In the case of egg donation by lavage, which is being used in the USA, policy commentators Sherman Elias and George Annas (1986, p. 65) feel that, 'legal control over the extracorporeal embryo should be vested in the sperm donor who has contributed genetically to it'. Neither identifiable mother is so deserving, neither the woman who conceives by AI nor the woman who will eventually receive the embryo and become pregnant if all goes as planned.

The American Fertility Society recommended that egg donation by uterine lavage continue to be tried out on women as a clinical experiment. In the most straightforward use of egg donation by lavage, a woman (called the 'egg donor') is inseminated with sperm from the male partner of the 'receiving' couple. If the woman conceives, the resulting embryo is 'washed out' of her womb before implantation, and then inserted into the woman whose partner had contributed the sperm. The American Fertility Society had reservations about the risks to the 'donor' woman of ectopic pregnancy. They also had reservations about the high risk of paternity uncertainty. They were afraid that the 'egg donor' woman might have sexual intercourse, and the resulting child might not be the genetic offspring of the man whose sperm was used for insemination! They are so worried about paternity uncertainty that they repeatedly suggest using medical tests to prove the genetic relationship between father and child.

Surrogacy

'Surrogate' motherhood, where a woman bears a child for another person or couple, is one of many procedures which emerged in conjunction with *in vitro* methods. Surrogacy raises a number of issues about social class and control of women, the meaning of pregnancy and childbirth, creating categories of motherhood, sale and exploitation of poor women and women in developing countries. In this book I do not address these issues in depth, but only touch on some of them. In this section I look at the responses to surrogacy by some government committees and the American Fertility Society, and examples of court cases.

Surrogacy was treated by government committees as much more problematic than IVF. Most Western European countries and Australian states have banned the practice, either formally or informally. However, most accept that private surrogacy arrangements between individuals are beyond their control. The surrogacy situation is different in North America. The practice is flourishing as a commercial enterprise in some states of the United States amidst a confusion of clashing legal opinions about it. *Newsweek* magazine reported in November 1985 that 600 surrogate babies had so far been born through commercial surrogacy transactions (Gelman and Shapiro, 1985). In Canada, the Ontario Law Reform Commission Report accepted surrogacy, proposing that surrogacy, like adoption, be controlled in the courts.

Neither disapproval nor approval of surrogacy in these government reports have been judgements based on women's autonomy and interests. Once again, government concern about surrogacy can be understood in terms of the wish to subordinate women's behaviour in the interests of the state and the ideology of the family.

For example, a majority of the British Warnock Committee recommended the criminalisation of commercial surrogacy arrangements, referring to the practice as 'recruitment of women' (p. 47), imitating the language of prostitution. But arguments against surrogacy which they cite are not about exploitation of women as reproductive commodities, but about the image of motherhood and woman's sexuality. The arguments they cite paint a disreputable picture of 'surrogate' mothers, calling them a 'third party' in marriage, saying the practice of surrogacy is 'inconsistent with human dignity', and that it distorts the mother–child relationship (pp. 44–5). The arguments taken together suggest that a woman who would become a 'surrogate mother' is either morally reprehensible or being asked by someone else to do wrong.

For the Warnock Committee, I would say, the problem with

accepting surrogacy as a medical treatment was that there is no respectable place for the 'carrying mother' in the ideology of motherhood, which portrays motherhood in strict terms as a natural, biological, inevitable, inviolable process. Surrogacy, another kind of motherhood, interferes most obviously with the concept of exclusivity within marriage. With the kinds of egg and sperm donation the Warnock Committee found acceptable, the third party (sperm and egg donors) will at least remain anonymous and remote.[3] A pregnant woman is more difficult to cover up, especially since she might change her mind and wish to keep the child she had agreed to give up.

The Warnock Committee is not concerned for women, but for motherhood's image. They do not feel the need to protect women from being asked to donate eggs, a potentially exploitative action as the Victoria Waller Committee acknowledged. Medical science is allowed to ask women for body parts (eggs, follicular fluid, placenta) for research. Yet, since 'no woman ought to be asked' (p. 45) to be a surrogate mother, accept the risks and give up a child, the state will protect women by banning the practice of surrogacy. Outright evidence of the Warnock Committee's lack of concern for women can be read in their view on private surrogacy arrangements. They suggest that private surrogacy arrangements should not by criminalised, not in order to protect women, but 'as we are anxious to avoid children being born to mothers subject to the taint of criminality' (p. 47).

When ethical committees address the possible exploitation of women as surrogate mothers, they see other women as the most blameworthy exploiters of all. The Warnock, Ontario and American Fertility Society Reports explicitly mention exploitation of 'carrying mothers' by other women who might not want to go through pregnancy. Husbands who might desire genetic offspring are not mentioned as potential exploiters, yet the most common kind of surrogacy occurs by insemination of the 'carrying mother' with sperm from the male partner of the couple who will receive the child. A husband's desire to have his own genetic offspring is never evaluated in such negative terms. In fact it is respected, even if it poses risks to women, as in the case of IVF for treatment of subfertility in men.

Despite banning, private surrogacy arrangements may occur, and this prompted government committees to ponder the question, who should be considered the mother in such cases? The Warnock

Report proposed that in the event the question of maternity should arise, the woman who bears the child and gives birth should be considered the mother. The Victoria Waller Report explicitly stated that in all cases the woman who carries the child is the mother, whether or not her egg ('genetic material') is used. She then may relinquish her rights to an adopting couple. (The Warnock Report's recommendation that the woman who bears the child should always be considered the mother is not the final decision on the matter. In their 1986 consultation paper on IVF issues, the Department of Health and Social Security raised the question of maternity identity again, asking for public opinion on the Warnock Report recommendation.)

By contrast, both the Ontario Law Reform Commission and the Ethics Committee of the American Fertility Society recommended that a surrogacy contract should be legally binding, and that the courts should identify the contracting couple as the legal parents. Thus, the woman who bears the child would not be considered the mother at birth. The implications of such a recommendation are astounding, suggesting that women who give birth can be divided into two categories, those who are considered the mother, and those who are not. This is a controversial decision, however. US policy commentators Sherman Elias and George Annas (1986) recommended that the 'gestational mother' should have first rights to the born child, just as in the Victoria Waller Report.

The Ontario Law Reform Commission added that a binding surrogacy contract should include specifics about 'prenatal restrictions upon the surrogate mother's activities before and after the conception, including dietary obligations; and . . . conditions under which prenatal screening of the child may be justified or required, for example, by ultrasound, fetoscopy or amniocentesis' (p. 284). US surrogacy agencies already draw up contracts which command women to behave in a particular way during pregnancy, to abstain from smoking and drinking, to undergo certain compulsory medical tests during the pregnancy, and so on. As many lawyers have pointed out, regulation of a surrogate mother's behaviour is setting standards for 'correct' maternal behaviour, and the possibility of extending *legal control* with respect to these 'standards' to all pregnant women. (This kind of legal control is an extension of the kind of control of women in the name of 'fetal neglect' which I discussed in Chapter 2.)

The Ontario Law Reform Commission recommended that

surrogacy be controlled by the courts, while the Ethics Committee of the American Fertility Society recommended that surrogacy be considered a 'clinical experiment' to assess it. There are two extremely important points to make here.

First, that surrogacy as a medical 'therapy', controlled by the medical profession or the courts, is harmful to women, as illustrated by the surrogacy contract situation. It further removes control of pregnancy and childbirth from women; it defines women with respect to our breeding capacity. This is not about women's right to control our own bodies. Even though the 1985 Surrogacy Arrangements Act in Britain made any *commercial* surrogacy transaction a criminal offence, this is not necessarily enough to protect women. Many doctors and IVF practitioners, including Edwards and Steptoe, would accept surrogacy as a womb-for-therapy, that is under the control of medical science (see Chapter 4).

The second point follows. Egg donation and surrogacy, whether accepted or banned, have perplexed the regulation-makers on the status of motherhood. Because of egg donation, embryo donation and surrogacy, *they* now recognise 'genetic mother', 'biological mother', 'carrying mother', 'social mother'. *They* have split women up into new categories of motherhood. They now ponder questions such as, what is the status of a woman who agrees to be a 'surrogate' mother by receiving an IVF embryo created with another woman's egg? Is the mother the woman who contributes *genetically* to the child, or the woman who bears the child and gives birth? Such a question infers that the 'biological' aspect of women's role in reproduction could be reduced to that of 'egg donor'. These technology-created categories of motherhood and their possible codification in law are a horrific denial of women's integrity, of the realities of pregnancy and birth. Clearly, the woman who labours and gives birth is the mother.

On 30 March 1987 a repressive precedent was set in the USA, in what had become known as the 'Baby M' case. In the state of New Jersey, Judge Sorkow ordered Mary Beth Whitehead to give her baby up to William and Elizabeth Stern. Mary Beth Whitehead had agreed to carry a baby for the Sterns, but had changed her mind about giving the baby up. The Sterns took her to court. Through the Infertility Center of New York, the Sterns had made the surrogacy contract with Mary Beth Whitehead, who agreed to be inseminated with William Stern's sperm and carry a child for them. After giving birth, Mary Beth Whitehead gave the baby over to the Sterns, but she decided she could not accept the US$10000 fee. A few days after, she asked to keep the child. A long scenario ensued which ended in a court battle where Judge Sorkow ruled that the Sterns should take custody of the child. It was apparent that the judgement was made, not only on the legality of a surrogacy contract *per se*, but also because the middle-class Sterns were considered better able than the working-class Whiteheads to provide for the child materially, socially, and morally. Most significantly, Judge Sorkow also claimed that because the child was genetically related to William Stern, 'He cannot purchase what is already his' (Arditti, 1987). In an article in *Science for the People*, Rita Arditti (1987, p. 23) commented on the case. By this twisted logic, she wrote, the child has only one parent, the father.

> Surrogacy reinforces the patriarchal view that the woman is just a container, an incubator of the man's sperm. She receives it and gives it back as his baby . . . The term 'surrogate mother' is a misnomer, reflecting the male perspective that pervades this whole issue . . . the surrogacy agreement, the media, and all of the literature on this subject always call her a 'surrogate mother', while referring to the sperm donor as the 'natural father'. (see note at end of chapter)

In an earlier case, reported in *American Medical News* (1986), a judge in Detroit ruled that a couple who are the genetic parents of a child carried by a 'surrogate mother' are the legal parents of the child. Thus, the pregnant woman's relationship to the child she carries was considered secondary. That decision infers that genes (egg and sperm) are more significant than the labour and experience of a woman who becomes pregnant and gives birth, yet another example of the way 'genetic identity' is becoming socially important as a significant measure of human relationships.

In a 1987 case in Britain, the court did rule in favour of a woman who had contracted in a private arrangement to carry a child for a couple. She, like Mary Beth Whitehead, changed her mind and wanted to keep the twins she gave birth to. The court ruled in her favour, but based on the legal principle, 'the best interests of the child'. This illustrates my point about the nature of the 'best interests of the child' principle being used in the courts. Although the outcome of the decision is welcome the reasoning behind it is precarious for women. It leaves the opportunity for the courts to decide in surrogacy cases if the woman who gives birth is 'fit' to be the mother. Such judgements made by men of law in favour of the 'natural mother' have traditionally been informed by a notion of a strict biological mother–child bond, a 'natural' (passive, not active) mother–child relationship. This notion again fits a patriarchal definition of motherhood. It does not guarantee the recognition of women as human subjects, nor the unique contexts within which each woman makes life decisions about the care of children.

This issue of 'maternity identity' being debated by 'experts' is one of immediate importance for women. The final decision to keep a child or to give it up must always rest with the woman who gives birth, no matter what previous arrangements are made between her and others. The woman who goes through pregnancy and gives birth is the mother.

The empowerment of research science

The Warnock Report discussed applications of IVF methods on women; they discussed artificial insemination, egg donation, embryo donation, surrogacy, sex selection, and freezing eggs and embryos. They finally addressed the question of IVF-related research in the very last chapters of their report.

The Warnock Committee, like the other government committees discussed in this chapter, accepted a scientific meaning of reproduction without the least consideration that IVF-related research is experimentation on women. The ethics of using adult women for experimentation was not at issue, yet experimentation on *in vitro* embryos and clinical use of IVF cannot happen without experimentation using women's bodies.

The Warnock Report addressed the question of 'human embryo research' in terms of the embryo, not women. The main objections raised in the Report concerned the humanity of embryos and the fear of out-of-control scientists (the Frankenstein image). The Warnock Committee concluded that the embryo is not accorded the same status as a living person in English Law. From this a majority voted in favour of human embryo research, subject to restrictions, up to fourteen days after fertilisation *in vitro*. They never once mentioned that women's bodies are needed to gain access to eggs, tissue, and bodily fluids for embryo experiments; that women had been used as experimental subjects in IVF programmes years before the birth of the first baby conceived by IVF; and that women are the future experimental subjects of the research. Further, an entire section of the report addressed 'possible future developments in research' using *in vitro* embryos. Many of these projects have nothing whatsoever to do with infertility treatment. Possible future developments included genetic research and the development of methods for eugenic applications.

By accepting a scientific meaning of reproduction, government reports on IVF accepted the scientific view that genetic technology is necessary for healthy reproduction. They accepted genetics as a fact of reproductive practice without even discussing the meaning of modern genetics, its eugenic underpinnings, or the motivations of scientists.

When considering the acceptability of 'human embryo' research, the Ontario Law Reform Commission did acknowledge an 'ethical dilemma'. They recognised a potential clash between the requirements of researchers for body parts and 'ethical considerations relating to the control over one's body' (pp. 90–1). They suggested that one way to approach the issue is to deal with gametes (egg and sperm) as legal property by assuming that the person who produces the 'genetic material' owns it. This is a particularly legalistic approach. US lawyer Lori Andrews (1986) also espouses that people should be granted the right to treat our body parts as personal property, and she sees this as providing 'a framework for handling evolving issues regarding the control of extracorporeal biological materials', such as women's eggs for research purposes (p. 37).

The rationale that we 'own' our body parts, and that our body parts belong to us like commodities, is a price of the dualistic mind/body thinking that is so pervasive in Western culture. It serves the interests of medical researchers and for-profit clinics (see Corea, 1985). It legitimises exploitation on many fronts. Against this claim that we 'own' our body parts, Maria Mies and other feminists of the Beitrage zur Feministischen Theorie und Praxis wrote:

> If my belly (abdomen), my uterus and my ovaries are my private property then I'm allowed to sell or rent them. However, the

women's movement and in particular the women's health
movement has insisted that we do not possess our bodies, but that
we *are* our bodies (Our Bodies Ourselves). (Hanmer, 1986,
p. 10)

This seems to me the most empowering way to regard ourselves.

Why a radical stance

Some women believe that IVF and the other technologies of
reproduction and genetics could be liberating to us, if they were
controlled by women and used in women's interests. It is true that
reproductive technologies are potentially disruptive to patriarchal
ideology. IVF conceptions shake its foundations: 'natural' motherhood, kinship and the 'natural' nuclear family. Indeed this is why
IVF and the new reproductive technologies are defined and used in
a specific framework – within marriage, as a 'better' alternative to
adoption, controlled by the state in concert with medical scientists
to guarantee the continuation of traditional norms. However, the
subversive element of artificial reproduction technology does not
work in women's favour, even if women control it. If IVF were
taken to its 'logical' subversive end, it would change the balance of
power from the traditional dominant authorities of patriarchy *to a
new dominating authority, the technocrats.*

IVF and other new reproductive technologies are in either case
the inventions of the natural sciences and the biotechnology
industry brought to medicine. They are in either case eugenic, and
incorporate racist and ableist values (some genes/traits are better
than others, traits can be 'matched'). They are in either case sexist.
IVF, egg donation, embryo donation, surrogacy, genetic therapy,
genetic analysis of embryos and fetuses require women in the
service of 'experts' in scientific reproduction. The few examples
which appear to be positive benefits of IVF and genetic engineering
are not possible without the social costs.

There already exist socially sanctioned power differences
between women and men, and between patient and doctor. With
sophisticated technologies come an extra dimension of power
differences, between those who invent specific technologies with
particular aims, and those on whom they are used. Those who

believe that IVF, artificial wombs, and genetic engineering can be used to make life better trust that scientists and the state will not abuse their authority over women's eggs, embryos, and bodies – not realising that such a view means women should exchange our body parts and reproductive role for 'progress'. Even if the unfettered used of the new artificial reproductive technologies should make husbands obsolete, women would be at the service to reproductive engineers at worst. Or perhaps some women, those deemed 'fit' to breed, would be put in a position of making eugenic decisions about which embryos to 'choose', which 'genes' to perpetuate.

IVF and related technologies can potentially disrupt the dominant social meaning of reproduction, *but not in women's interests*. They just will recategorise women. Make more categories of subordination. IVF, embryo flushing, egg and embryo donation, and surrogacy, splits motherhood up into new categories. Women are not defining ourselves, medical scientists are defining us. There are 'carrying mothers' ('surrogate mothers') and 'egg donor mothers' who are called biological mothers but not social mothers, and there are social mothers who are not biological mothers. The meaning of the new reproductive technologies cannot be rehabilitated in women's interests. Power and control over reproduction would still lie with technological 'experts' who know about women's eggs, embryos, wombs and genes. Power and control would still lie with 'experts' over the majority of women.

Note on the 'Baby M' case

On 3 February 1988, the New Jersey Supreme Court overturned the 1987 lower court decision validating surrogacy contracts, challenging the label 'surrogate' for the natural mother, and restoring Mary Beth Whitehead as the legal mother, although custody remains with the Sterns. See Janice G. Raymond (1988) 'In The Matter of Baby M: Rejudged', *Reproductive and Genetic Engineering*, vol. 1, no. 2.

9

Transforming reality

A place of struggle

Each generation of the women's movement, Maria Mies has said, must re-examine, reassess and respond to the situations in which we find ourselves. In our generation, we find ourselves up against the further development and application of reproductive and genetic technologies. As Jalna Hanmer (1986) has stressed since the 1970s, these technologies are about more than biological reproduction; they are about social relations.

Reproductive and genetic technologies serve many levels of social ordering and control, as evidenced in the preceding chapters:

— Technologies such as IVF, egg and embryo freezing and genetic 'therapy' (engineering) alienate women from our reproductive processes, placing them in the hands of outside 'experts'. Women's subjective knowledge and experiences of fertility, pregnancy, birth and motherhood is marginalised by the supremacy of 'objective' data supplied by ultrasound scanning,[1] experiments on embryos and fetuses maintained outside women's bodies, and so on.

In these scientific approaches to reproduction, women are no longer the central subject of human procreation, as exemplified by IVF practice where women are displaced by couples, by IVF embryos, by fetus-as-patient, and by the IVF practitioner as the 'test-tube' father/creator in charge of our eggs and embryos and wombs.

By contrast, the resurgence of midwifery and home birth in industrialised countries, and the desire of many women to take a less interventionist path during pregnancy and birth affirms a woman-centred, life-affirming experience of reproduction, an affirmation of women's physical integrity, the integrity of the mother–child relationship, and of pregnancy and childbirth as a personal, sexual, familial, communal experience. Healing and midwifery are ancient activities, predating modern science. The emergence of gynaecology, as feminist writers such as Mary Daly (1979) and Barbara Ehrenreich and Deirdre English (1979) have chronicled, was a conquest of male professionals over women healers and midwives, and their old-wives remedies.

But even as feminist awareness grows, even as movements towards a woman-controlled, less interventionist approach to pregnancy and birth has been happening in many Western countries, an overriding expansion of doctor-controlled technological reproduction is apparent within the medical profession. In the Netherlands, for instance, where the health care system has been up till the 1980s relatively less interventionist compared to many other Western countries, reproductive health care for women is now becoming more technological (Sevenhuijsen and de Vries, 1984).

Egg and embryo selling, and 'womb leasing' are on the threshold of a new reproductive industry, with new national and international markets for a new kind of traffic in women and women's body parts.

Poor women will be the most vulnerable to exploitation. In *Right Wing Women*, Andrea Dworkin (1983) incisively criticises the often heard argument that women who wish to sell our reproductive capacities are exercising free will in the market-place. She writes:

> The arguments as to the social and moral appropriateness of this new kind of sale simply reiterate the view of female will found in discussions of prostitution . . . Again, the state has constructed the social, economic, and political situation in which the sale of some sexual or reproductive capacity is necessary to the survival of women. (p. 182)

The export of Western contraceptive technology to developing countries in the name of 'development aid' is part of a global economic and population control. In Bangladesh, the organisation UBINIG (Policy Research for Development Alternative) was founded on the principle that technocratic concepts of development are dehumanising, that development is not equivalent to more technology:

> The concept of development should mean the development of the real living people and their conditions of living . . . determined by the relations of its members among themselves and their access to productive resources. The real development implies the change in these conditions. UBINIG believes that equitable distribution of wealth and productive resources is the first step towards that change. (UBINIG, undated)

Reproductive and genetic technologies serve eugenic ideals, specific to particular nations for their particular 'needs'. IVF and related procedures carry the promise that medical scientists can control the 'products' of reproduction in accord with social 'needs' to eliminate disability, handicap, and human traits deemed 'inferior'.

With the application of the NRT's, genetic considerations become more socially pervasive than ever before. The scientific preoccupation with 'genetic identity' and genetic relationship is incorporated into our everyday lives, becoming of central importance to the state in defining social relations. It is an imposition on people's consciousness of family ties and human relations, and yet another imposition on women's relationship to our own reproductive capacities.

The new reproductive technologies are a 'technical fix', that is unsolutions for problems which are rooted in social and economic relations, and most fundamentally in our relationship to science and technology. The 'technical fix' approach is not life-respecting, but an effort in biological control, whether IVF for infertility, or amniocentesis and selective abortion for congenital conditions such as cleft palate, or freezing embryos in anticipation of nuclear disasters, or rating fetuses for genetic endowment, or changing the genetic composition of fetuses and people in the name of 'therapy'.

Scientist-controlled, technological reproduction offers solutions, but not in ways to empower women – to make us more in control of our health and social circumstances. These technical solutions in the long term, overall are made at the expense of women's health and integrity. Women's struggle for sexual, reproductive, economic and social autonomy is undermined by the proliferation of a kind of reproduction which necessitates interference from the state and its institutions, especially medical science professionals.

The promises of technology as a means of future liberation of human beings is forever unfulfilled. New 'wonder' drugs such as interferon have yet to cure either the common cold or cancer, as was originally promised. Mechanical organs and artificial 'muscular systems' invented by scientists working in space programmes and on military research, promised as the answer to certain kinds of disability, have never been seriously considered for such applications. They were not invented to empower the disabled but to 'outdo human muscles' (Taylor, 1968. p. 82). In this century the propagation of hypertechnologies is the propagation of more pain and more death, not more health and more life. *More* people are starving, despite high-yield agricultural methods, whose results have brought draught in some areas of the world and food mountains in other areas. Industrial waste and air pollution continues to cause ill health and death, and it threatens the life of the entire planet, as does the continued use of nuclear technology. As for reproductive technologies, they were not invented to empower women. To paraphrase the journal *Nature* (1983), the aim of IVF and the new reproductive technologies are to improve, so to speak, on women.

The social and health problems which the new reproductive technologies are supposed to 'fix' can only be adequately addressed in women's interests by looking to the roots of the problems in the first place. Feminists are looking to social movements, especially the women's movement, as a force for the social and political change necessary to address these problems.

Rosalie Bertell is one such social activist who looks to women as a force for change. In *No Immediate Danger: Prognosis for a Radioactive Earth*, Bertell (1985) documented direct correlations between health problems and radioactive contamination. Among these are infertility, miscarriage, and birth handicaps. Bertell has been criticised by scientists who admire her work and rigorous research, but who believe she goes 'too far'. For example, one critic agrees that low levels of radiation in the environment damage the nuclei of cells which later may manifest itself as cancer; but she disagrees with Bertell that low-level radiation depresses the immune system (Kec, 1987). How can a scientist say on the one hand that cellular mechanisms are fundamental to a persons life processes, and then on the other hand recognise only *one* deleterious effect of damage to those fundamental cells?

My own frustration with this kind of criticism stems from experience. When I was suffering with a number of symptoms from chemical poisening (from acetonitrile, which is a cyanide, and from a xylene derivative), a famous allergist in the USA told me he could find nothing to show that I was experiencing a reaction from these chemicals. State-of-the-art blood tests showed nothing. It was only later that I was able to trust own judgement about what was happening to me, and later still that it became common knowledge that many workers in a variety of jobs were becoming extremely ill and disabled due to daily contact with toxic chemicals, for example plant workers in the computer industry. The point I am trying to make is that overestimating 'technical' medical knowledge is naive and unhelpful. The testimony of people's experience has a reality of its own.

On reproductive rights

After a first chorus of 'reproductive technologies give women more choice', there is the question of the meaning of these technologies. As Maria Mies (1987) asks, do they make women happier and freer?

We are learning that it is no longer adequate to pose our demands for freedom in terms of 'rights' and 'choice'. There can only be a limited awareness of choice in a world where women do not control our own reproduction, where medical scientists armed with technologies, impose some choices at the expense of others; where reproductive options and children are bought and sold like commodities; where many Black women and minority women in Western countries, and women in 'Third World' countries, are coerced into 'choosing' abortion, sterilisation, and dangerous contraceptives; where reproductive and genetic technologies *require* the physical and social subordination of women. Barbara Katz Rothman rephrases this, 'The question is not whether choices are constructed, but how they are constructed' (Rothman, 1984, p. 32).

One of the most important areas for feminist discussion has been brought up by women in the disability rights movement. In their articles in the feminist anthology *Test-Tube Women* (1984), Anne Finger and Marsha Saxton urge women to reassess our relationship to pre-natal screening and selective abortion.

Marsha Saxton points out that the rationale for pre-natal screening is provided by the assumption that the life of a disabled fetus [a potential disabled person] should be ended. She writes that as a disabled woman who supports pro-choice on the issue of abortion, she could not herself contemplate pre-natal screening during her own pregnancy because of this assumption.

Also writing as a disabled feminist, Anne Finger points to feminist accountability in this area, that the abortion rights movement has exploited the fears and stereotypes of disability. Saxton emphasises that the reproductive rights movement has not adequately acknowledged the sexuality of disabled women and the implications of pre-natal screening technology. As feminists, both Saxton and Finger support pro-choice on the issue of abortion, and they do not feel this is inconsistent with their disability rights politics.

Changing our relationship to genetic screening must include practical considerations – great social change – as well. In a presentation at the Women's Hearings on Reproductive and Genetic Technology at the European Parliament in Brussels in 1986, Theresia Degener said 'fear of the birth of a handicapped child is only too justified because for mothers it usually means isolation and discrimination, giving up their jobs, and/or poverty . . . Only too often these economic and social conditions are confused with the disability itself, by equating it with concepts such as "misery" and "despair".' Once understood in its social context, the kinds of changes needed become more obvious.

The social environment and social norms *en*able certain people, and *dis*able others. Finger urges the reproductive rights movement to incorporate the demands of disabled people for access, sexual freedom, and parental rights. Instead of focusing on fetal disability, she refocuses the discussion on the reproductive rights of disabled women and men.

This is an important issue for discussion and learning if we are to reject the politics of the 'lesser evil'. One woman's lesser evil (for example, eugenic abortion is better than no abortion rights) is another woman's oppression (a world where certain people are unwelcome and considered 'preventable', a world where disabled women are not considered sexual, that is not considered women at all). It is most important now with the expansion of eugenic technologies (genetic screening, genetic therapy) by the use of genetic engineering. As a group of Japanese women activists put it, 'The freedom of abortion which we demand requires inherently a struggle not only against the State and men but also against the eugenic ideal within women ourselves'.[2]

Feminist demands for adequate primary health care, a clean environment, and the social and economic conditions that respect women's health and the health of all children must come from a different philosophy than does eugenics.

Technology is not neutral

In *The Science Question in Feminism*, Sandra Harding (1986) delineates in particular what she and other feminist critics see as the male bias embedded in scientific thought, its objectivity, rationality, and disinterestedness. Rehabilitation or control of existing scientific theories is not enough; the feminist issue with science is to challenge *content* of scientific theories. This, it seems to me, is the obvious task once we acknowledge that science and technology are not neutral.

Yet, many social activists, including feminists, incorporate the 'technology is neutral' belief into a use/abuse analysis of reproductive technology. Those who adhere to the use/abuse argument believe that IVF technology is neutral and can be used for either good or for bad. So, a sensitive IVF advocate might argue that IVF is bad when it exploits women, or is restricted to heterosexual women living with men, but that IVF is good when women choose it 'freely' and are not discriminated against. Underlying presumptions of this point of view are that the pursuit of science ('biological facts') does not incorporate moral/political decisions, and that IVF and genetic engineering do not occur in a particular ideological context. But they do.

The use/abuse argument ignores the realities of IVF: the fact that what women go through is not considered (because if it were, the nature of the NRTs and experimentation on women would be revealed); the fact that thousands of women are experimented with to make IVF happen; the fact that 'spare' embryos for research come from administering superovulatory drugs to women, and carrying out other biochemical and physiological manipulations of women's healthy life processes; the fact that the existence of IVF and its correlative technologies pre-empts other, non-technological choices; the fact that NRTs are fundamentally eugenic; the fact that IVF further pathologises all aspects of women's reproduction; the fact that the dissociation of women's reproduction from our sensuous selves changes our relationship to reproduction, making it further out-of-women's-control; the fact that women's bodies are being exploited for commercial markets; the interplay of genetic engineering, reproductive engineering and the whole area of biotechnology; and the fact that, as Sultana Kamal (1987) stresses, reproductive technology is for Western women what contraceptive technology has been for most of the women in 'Third World' countries, that is, a population control plan from 'experts' that use women for racist, eugenic ends.

The common denominator of reproductive technolgy, whether hightech or lowtech, new or old, in the clinical setting or in the laboratory, is a scientific approach to women's reproduction. This approach imposes an aggressive, confrontational relationship to nature, in this case to women's reproduction. It down-plays reproductive rituals *and up-plays life risks* other than those the technology makes. So, if a woman refuses to undergo Caeserean section birth the doctor orders, it is seen as a woman taking a risk; but the incredible risk to women of IVF and other technological procedures are dismissed by government inquiries and IVF practitioners as minor risks.

Scientific control of 'human reproduction' requires that some women be posed as 'Other', as the clinical and laboratory object of study for the scientist–observer. Such an approach could only proceed in social conditions which allow them. If scientists asked different kinds of questions about biology, if medical scientists recognised women as the active social subjects of reproduction, not as passive breeders, if they respected women's reproductive freedom and autonomy, then they would not be pursuing IVF and human embryo research.

A few generations ago, the technologies of modern physics were incorporated into our lives. Many nuclear physicists believed that the laws of energy and matter were not only of utmost importance to 'pure' knowledge, but also to commerce and industry, wealth and poverty, to political and social systems. Today, biological principles about living matter deployed as genetic engineering and reproductive engineering are similarly being incorporated into every level of life by technocrats, those doctors, scientists, technologists and industrialists who believe that the laws of the life sciences should touch the whole human experience, from the food we eat, to health care, to the way we reproduce. This is the meaning of biotechnology.

The new reproductive and genetic technologies are as potent an area of scientific hegemony as nuclear technology has been. If you look at the history of nuclear fission ('splitting of the atom') next to the evolution of the new reproductive/genetic technologies, the parallel is unmistakable. The development of nuclear technology for bombs and for energy came out of the development of 'basic' research in particle physics; it unlocked possibilities 'at variance with all previous experience'; it gave men the capability to 'control' matter on a larger scale than ever before; despite recognising the most horrific possibilities, scientists felt, as C. P. Snow said, 'There is no ethical problem; if the invention is not prevented by physical laws, it will certainly be carried out somewhere in the world'; the nuclear invention prompted government committees to investigate it, and seek to 'control' it; and as C. P. Snow predicted in 1939, 'We have seen too much of human selfishness and frailty to pretend that men can be trusted with a new weapon of gigantic power.'[3]

Today, a new scientific generation is taking a similar path with reproductive/genetic technologies. The technologies are to a large extent the products of so-called basic research in embryology and genetics; the NRTs give 'experts' the power to alter the biological make-up of all living things, including people, and the course of evolution. Gene and embryo manipulation is most certainly an entirely new situation, 'at variance with all previous experience' brought to us by enthusiastic, hopeful scientists who plead a case that their technologies are benign. The NRTs are as certainly 'a new weapon of gigantic power'. And who can trust men with such gigantic power this time around?

There have been strong, vocal criticisms of science and technology from many sectors, on the pupulist level from environmentalists and the peace movement, from professionals such as Doctors Against Nuclear Arms, from the US-based Science for the People, and the British Society for Social Responsibility in Science. The Green parties in Western Europe have gathered together the issues of peace, sex equality, ecology and exploitation of the 'Third World', calling for a devolution from nation states to a fundamental restructuring of societies. Environmental groups have been fighting against the use of genetic engineered organisms and products. In the USA, the Foundation on Economic Trends has persistently filed law suits in order to delay the release of genetic engineered organisms into the open environment. Jeremy Rifkin, director of the Foundation on Economic Trends, espouses a fundamental change in the way we live in the world. Rifkin's point is that the high-tech road is insecure and dangerous despite the (unfulfilled) promises of social and economic security for all, and the promises of 'deterence'. A love affair with technology is ultimately destructive, and only an empathetic relationship with nature (the environment) will bring true security (Rifkin, 1985).

A growing number of feminists have taken the criticisms to a radical level, making the links between reproductive technologies and other patriarchal manifestations of technology, such as nuclear technology. Feminist ecologist Sarah Jansen (1986) suggests why: 'Our alienation, our dissatisfaction, means that we are far more radical than the male critics in our search for the subjective quality of science and technology and for alternatives'. And so it has been. In *The Biological Time Bomb* Gordon Rattray Taylor (1986) warns that the costs of the revolution in biology – its technology – are terrifyingly high. And although he makes a strong case for the view that knowledge is not neutral, although he believes that certain kinds of knowledge should not be pursued, although he believes that technology is to blame, he carefully concludes that 'There will have to be a biological "ice-box" in which the new techniques can be placed until society is ready for them' (p. 21).

Feminist critics of the new technologies reject that conclusion. We understand that the new 'techniques' can only be understood in the social context in which they were invented. 'Technical' techniques such as IVF exist in the context of a whole technology of reproduction which also includes egg and embryo freezing, superovulation of women, artificial wombs, genetic selection of embryos, genetic engineering, and more. We understand that the scientific approach to reproduction via high technologies is 'logical' in a world where women's bodies are considered exploitable. We understand that this world view can only exist in sexist cultures, a contemporary affront to women's human integrity. As Janice Raymond (1987) writes, for women to be valued, 'women's bodies must have the same freedom from intervention, intrusion, and invasion as men's' (p. 65).

Towards a feminist ethic

In *Science and Gender* (1984) Ruth Bleier places the feminist challenge: 'Having defined the problem as nothing less than an enveloping patriarchal consciousness and a more than 4000-year-old patriarchal civilization that has ordered social behaviours, forms of social organization and systems of thought, including science, how can we view the possibilities and directions for change?' (p. 199). Bleier sees feminist visions of a new science and technology as part of the whole of the women's movement, 'a revolutionary movement in thought and behaviour so profound and so rooted in a transformed counsciousness that it will not stop until all Western consciousness and civilization are transformed' (p. 199).

Feminist resistance to the new reproductive technologies is not a negative stance, but a positive one, where we can re-assert *women's* power and knowledge and experience *to ask our own questions* about fertility, fertility problems, childbirth, childrearing, motherhood, abortion. The women's health movement, reproductive rights activists, feminist historians and critics of the new technologies, while demystifing the politics behind the myth that reproductive technology is neutral, are fighting for this. Feminism seeks a world where women's lives will be different. While resisting eugenic technologies, we can explore what other kinds of research and medical approaches will serve women's needs.

Maria Mies sets out some of the changes that must be made in our thinking and our actions in 'Why Do We Need All This? A Call Against Genetic Engineering and Reproductive Technology' (1987). Positive response is twofold. First, refuse to be defeatist, and actively protest against the proliferation of reproductive and genetic engineering in both 'First World' and 'Third World' countries. Second, we can continue to look for alternatives to address women's needs.

Concerning the first kind of response, social protest is the power base for change. Industrialised nations are locked into a dependent relationship with science and technology. The power of technology is everywhere and the interests of the privileged are tied up in it, and not only in the arena of industry and commerce. The world view which embraces technology is also the most credible in almost every academic discipline. It is not easy to give up Rationality (so-called, in my view). IVF practitioners in the universities are protected by the 'academic freedom' principle. So, resistance must take the shape of community organising and local protesting, debate over what these issues mean for the women on whom they are used, exposing acitivities going on in our backyards, calling for public accountability on these issues, and demanding our right as individuals and communities to say 'no' to these technologies.

A women-centred approach to reproduction recognises the interrelationship among oppressions, among sexism, racism, ableism, class division. It recognises economic and global inequalities at play in our dependency on technologies. It means we must accept that everything is not solvable by some technical solution, and admit that there are risks to living that 'experts' cannot solve for us. It means that the most privileged women must give things up. Gross consumerism in one part of the world means exlpoitation of women in another.

One feminist response to the NRTs is the international information network, FINRRAGE (Feminist international Network of Resistance to Reproductive Technology and Genetic Engineering), which I mentioned in the Introduction to this book.[4] Women are taking part in the network to share information on what is happening in all our countries, and lending support to local, national and international campaigns against the NRTs.

At the Emergency Conference on the New Reproductive Technologies in Sweden, in 1985, the visions of many of these women from different countries transformed my own feelings of powerlessness into strength for thinking more positively about resisting the NRTs. One was a talk by feminist writer and engineer Pat Hynes (1987). She used as a model environmental protection legislation in the USA, basing her approach on the belief that women have a civil right to live unendangered. One approach she considers is the concept of acceptable or allowable risk. Applied to the new reproductive technologies, women could demand that there be established an acceptable level risk *before* these procedures are allowed to be used on women.

In searching for alternatives to patriarchal science, Sarah Jansen set out a basic agenda: to create a sense of wholeness, to suspend the separation between subject and object, that 'protective shield' of scientists. This is not a romantic holism, but rather a bringing together again of our living and working experiences. Jansen suggests that the use of 'technical' techniques in reproduction should be compatible with reproductive practices and rituals. Tapping the power of the non-technical should have a quite different effect from violent techniques which are dissociated from the underlying reasons for the problems they are supposedly trying to solve, and so can only aim to 'break the bodies resistance' (Jansen, 1986). I would say that IVF and genetic engineering technologies are examples of techniques which attempt to 'break the bodies resistance', while fertility awareness learning groups and self-help groups offer women ways of acquiring more information about alternatives to high technologies and coming to terms with fertility problems. There is infinite room to grow.[5]

At the Third International Interdisciplinary Congress on Women in Dublin in 1987, Alison Solomon talked about her own experiences of infertility as a life crisis, and her ideas of a two-pronged feminist approach to it.[6] This would entail immediate help on a personal level, in the form of counselling aimed to support the woman, to 'be with the woman' as Solomon puts it, to allow space to explore her feelings and deal with the crisis. In tandem with this individual support, feminists must also deal with the social stigma of infertility, as this dimension is of utmost significance. There will always be cases of women who are not able to bear a child. 'Technical' solutions to fertility problems do not solve the social pressures women experience with respect to fertility, motherhood, and biological parenthood.

I will end on the note on which I began this book, because it continues to impress on me. To change our relationship to science and technology in the most woman-respecting, life-respecting way, we must start from the recognition that *we are our bodies, we are ourselves*. We do not have to accept the man-made paradoxes and the splitting up of women into parts (eggs, embryos, wombs, placenta) which has been so ingrained as to seem natural. We can overturn the dualities of mind/body, rational/emotional, science (what men do)/not science (what women do), and the ancient conceptual split embryo/woman. Knowledge of women's fertility and procreative powers must have to do with our bodies, and be grounded in experiences in the world, in feeling and doing (which also includes thinking and observing), not what scientists find out for us in laboratories after they have taken our insides out. Mainstream scientists' 'out there' is our 'here and now'.

Appendix

What's what: medical/science organisations in Great Britain mentioned in this book

The British Medical Association is the representative body for medical doctors. Their journal, *The British Medical Journal*, is a forum for all doctors and physicians, and allows a wide range of medical opinion.

The Medical Research Council (MRC) is the main source of public funding for medical research in Britain. The MRC also operates and supports several research facilities throughout the country. Medical research includes basic biological research as well as clinical research.

The Lancet is the most prestigious general medical journal in Britain. In the USA *The New England Journal of Medicine* is comparable.

Nature is a British science journal of international scope. It has been called the most famous science journal in the world. It addresses the entire range of scientific topics in editorials, news reports and research papers. It is a platform for the latest developments in science and a forum for the science community. It is a mouthpiece for the scientific establishment in Britain.

The Royal College of Obstetricians and Gynaecologists (RCOG) is the main organisation of these specialists, with the most power in representing their interests.

The Royal Society is the scientific body in Britain comparable to national academies of science in other countries. It was founded in 1660, one of the first bodies devoted to the new 'natural philosphy'.

The Voluntary Licensing Authority (VLA) was set up by the MRC and RCOG to oversee the practice of IVF (*in vitro* fertilisation, the 'test-tube'

194

baby procedure) and related research on human embryos. It was formed along the lines which the Warnock Committee recommended, as a temporary measure until the government authorised a statutory licensing authority. Although it is voluntary, most IVF practitioners in Britain have said they abide by its guidelines. The VLA held its first meeting on 26 March 1985. For information write to The VLA Secretariat, 20 Park Crescent, London W1N 4AL.

The Warnock Report (published in 1984) is the Report of the Committee of Inquiry into Human Fertilisation and Embryology, requested by the Government of Great Britain in 1982 to examine the social, ethical and legal implications of developments in the field of 'human assisted reproduction' (IVF and related issues). It takes its name from the chair of the inquiry, Baroness Mary Warnock. Committees of Inquiry are *ad hoc* advisory bodies technically appointed by the British Crown, whose function is to report on some socially urgent matter on which new legislation seems desirable. The Warnock committee prompted other European governments to set up similar committees of their own. It is available as *A Question of Life* (1985) by Mary Warnock.

Glossary

Amniocentesis A pre-natal test performed after the fourteenth week of pregnancy, usually not before the sixteenth week, used to diagnose certain fetal abnormalities. The procedure carries risks and errors in diagnosis may occur. The pregnant woman is given a local anaesthetic and a needle is inserted through the abdominal wall and into her womb. A sample of amniotic fluid which surrounds the fetus is withdrawn, cultured and analysed to detect certain chromosome, gene and biochemical abnormalities. Chromosome analysis detects the sex of the fetus.

Artificial insemination: AI A simple procedure by which sperm is deposited in a woman's vagina as close to the cervix as possible. AID designates artificial insemination by donor sperm; AIH designates homologous insemination or artificial insemination using the husband's sperm. Many women simply use the term 'insemination' or 'self-insemination' to describe the practice.

Artificial womb The development of a human fetus outside a woman's womb, under laboratory conditions. Also called ectogenesis.

Biotechnology The exploitation of biochemical sources and technologies to create products and methods for industry, medicine, and the military.

Blastocyst A mammalian embryo at the first stage in development, formed after division of the fertilised egg.

Chorionic villi sampling: CVS A relatively new pre-natal screening procedure for analysis of fetal tissue. A small amount of chorion tissue surrounding the fetus is removed through the pregnant woman's cervix. It is performed at eight to fourteen weeks of pregnancy, and results can be evaluated overnight. Preliminary studies show it carries a greater risk of miscarriage than amniocentesis, and other attendant risks have yet to be determined. There has been variable success in obtaining villi for analysis, and a greater risk of error in diagnosis (see Ridler and Grewal, 1984).

Chromosomes Thread-like structures in the nucleus of a cell where **genes**

are packaged. In human beings each body cell contains 46 chromosomes: 22 matched pairs and a pair of sex chromosomes. **Sex chromosomes** operate in the biological sex-determining processes of a species. In humans, as in most animals, there are two kinds of sex chromosomes, the X chromosome and the Y chromosome. A combination of two X chromosomes gives a female, while one X and one Y gives a male (but several variations of these two combinations do exist, e.g. an XYY combination in a small number of males). The sex chromosomes carry many genes, some related to biological sex characteristics, and others unrelated to sex. Thus, there is a tendency for certain inherited disorders to occur more frequently in one sex if the genes occur on a sex chromosome. These conditions are called *sex linked* disease. Haemophilia, which primarily effects males, is an example.

Clone Genetically identical organisms. They are produced from a single individual by asexual reproduction, that is without union of egg and sperm. In mammals, clones can be produced by **nucleus substitution** or by **embryo division**. Cells and genes can also be cloned.

Congenital condition Congenital means present at birth, and so congenital conditions are those present in a baby at birth. They are not necessarily inherited (genetic); and some conditions triggered by environmental factors may mimic genetic disorders (and thus be incorrectly diagnosed as genetic disease). Congenital illnesses occur in varying degrees of seriousness. Congenital conditions may be due to (i) chromosomal differences (e.g. Down's Syndrome, most cases of which are not inherited but occur in a particular pregnancy by 'random mutation'); (ii) an inherited gene (e.g. sickle cell anaemia); (iii) injury or infectious diseases during pregnancy (e.g. Rubella); (iv) environmental factors such as drugs (e.g. thalidomide), chemicals (e.g. dioxin), and radioactive contamination; (v) combinations of hereditary and environmental factors. These categories are not fixed in that hereditary and environmental factors are always intertwined.

Cytogenetics The study of genetic inheritance in relation to the structure and function of cells.

DNA: Deoxyribonucleic acid The molecule that makes up the genetic material of most living organisms. Genes are units of DNA. (The term 'gene' predates the discovery in 1953 of DNA).

DNA fingerprinting or genetic fingerprinting A technique which enables an individual's unique set of genes to be printed on an X-ray film. It can be used on a blood sample, or other bodily fluid or tissue. The resulting 'genetic profile' can be used to match an individual with the blood sample, and it can be used to establish familial relationship, especially paternity and maternity. The method was developed at Leicester University by British geneticist Aleca Jeffreys, and is being commercialised by the chemical company ICI. It has been used in Britain for police work and in immigration cases.

Down's Syndrome   (Trisomy 21) Individuals with an extra chromosome no. 21 are born with this condition, where there are characteristic physical features and a greater susceptability to certain medical disorders. Severity of the condition varies. Physical therapy benefits many people with the condition.

Embryo   Commonly, the early stages of development before recognisable human features are formed, at about eight weeks or so. Scientific usage varies.

Embryo division   Splitting of an embryo outside the female body (an *in vitro* embryo) at an early stage when each section may continue development; thus it may result in multiple copies of the original single embryo, and is considered a form of cloning.

Embryo flushing   The procedure of 'washing out' a fertilised egg from a woman's womb before implantation takes place. Also called **surrogate embryo transfer, uterine lavage,** or **lavage.**

Embryo replacement: ER   A method used in conjunction with IVF treatment, in which the doctor inserts an *in vitro* embryo into the womb of the same woman whose egg is used.

Embryo transfer: ET   The procedure in which the doctor inserts an embryo into a woman's womb. The embryo can be an IVF embryo or an embryo flushed from a woman's womb before implantation occurs. The woman who receives it might be the same woman whose egg is used, or she might be a second woman, who did not contribute her own egg to the embryo. (Some IVF practitioners use the term ET when two different women are involved; some do not make that distinction, and use ET to mean any embryo insertion into a woman's womb.)

Embryo twinning   Embryo division in which the embryo is split into two identical embryos.

Endometriosis   A painful condition of the female reproductive system in which the lining of the womb is found sticking to other organs in the woman's body. It often leads to fertility problems (of varying degrees).

Estrogen   A collective term for a group of naturally occurring hormones with a variety of functions, for example it is necessary to complete the development (maturing) of eggs during a woman's menstrual cycle. Synthetic estrogens are drugs produced in laboratories which are similar in chemical structure to naturally occurring estrogens, but not identical. Their function is to alter or interfere with the production of menstrual cycle hormones.

Eugenics The science of the improvement of the human species by genetic means championed by Sir Francis Galton (1822--1911) who proposed the idea of improving physical and mental characteristics by selective parenthood.
Negative eugenics aims to decrease the propagation of certain types (e.g. the handicapped). The term is used today to describe selective abortion of fetuses with certain conditions. **Positive eugenics** aims to increase the propagation of 'desirable' human types. In medical science, it denotes an approach whereby genetic disorders can be remedied or averted, e.g. by sperm selection, egg selection or genetic engineering. See **gene therapy.**

Fetus Commonly, the developing embryo which has achieved recognisable human features, about eight weeks onward in humans. Scientific usage varies.

Follicle An enclosing cluster of cells that protects and nourishes a structure within. In women, follicles in the ovaries surround the developing egg. Follicular fluid, which encases the developing egg within the follicle, is an often-used component in IVF research and practice.

Frozen embryo Early embryos placed in serum and a 'cryoprotectant' (chemical that protects the embryo from being damaged at low temperatures) can be frozen in liquid nitrogen, at a temperature of $-196F$. In 1987, there were a reported 10000 frozen embryos in storage around the world.
A technique also exists now for freezing women's eggs. The long-term effects of the freezing procedures on human embryos and women's eggs are unknown.

Gamete A sex cell, either an egg (ovum, oocyte) or sperm (spermatozoon). In human beings, each gamete contains 23 chromosomes, half the number to make up a full set of chromosomes. When an egg and sperm fuse at fertilisation, a full set of 46 chromosomes results. In contrast to gametes are all the other cells in the body (called somatic cells) which contain 46 chromosomes in their nuclei.

Gene A segment of DNA which carries genetic information. In human beings they are (mostly) packaged in chromosomes in the nuclei of cells. Before the discovery of DNA, genes were described as 'units of heredity'. The DNA in egg and sperm carry genetic information from one generation to the next. From the molecular point of view, DNA plays a basic role in embryo development and body growth and maintenance.

Gene analysis DNA is removed from cells, spliced into pieces, and the pieces are then separated from one another and analysed. In principle, genes associated with diseases may be identified directly with 'gene probes', or indirectly by comparing fetal DNA with the DNA of genetic relations.
A 'gene probe' is a sequence of DNA which 'recognises' the same

sequence among the DNA being analysed. It works by a process called complementary pairing. When a gene for a condition is 'found', it can be cloned and modified for use as a probe. Gene probes have been produced for a sickle cell anaemia, phenylketonuria, beta thalassaemia, and more. In 1987, researchers 'found' the gene for a rare form of cleft palate, and predicted that a gene probe could soon be available.

Gene therapy   Genetic engineering techniques applied to humans in order to alter or replace 'defective' genes. 'Gene therapy' may also be directed at human embryos and fetuses, whether the woman is pregnant or whether the embryos/fetuses are maintained outside her body. The procedures are experimental, but the proponents believe they can be developed to prevent or treat certain genetic disorders.

Genetic engineering   The use of experimental techniques to change the characteristics of an organism by altering its DNA (i.e. its genes). Genetic engineering is an all-embracing term for several techniques some of which involve manipulation on the level of the cell (e.g. **cloning**), and some of which involve manipulation on the level of the DNA itself (e.g. 'gene manipulation').
'Gene manipulation' is the use of techniques to isolate and manipulate genes on the molecular level. By this method, pieces of the DNA (genes) can be removed from the cell; the pieces can then be analysed or inserted into another organism's DNA. If all goes as planned an inserted gene will carry out its function in the new organism. For example, human genes for making human growth hormone have been incorporated into the bacteria E.coli; the bacteria then become living 'factories' for the manufacture of human growth hormone. Gene manipulation is considered the most promising of genetic engineering methods for commercial, medical, and military use. It allows scientists to insert genes into an organism where they do not naturally occur. It is the basis of **gene therapy** and new **genetic screening** diagnostic tests.

Genetics   The science aimed at understanding what genes are and how they work.

Genetic screening   The use of diagnostic tests to acquire genetic or partly genetic information about an individual. Such tests can be used (i) on adults to test if they are 'carriers' of genetic disease; (ii) on pregnant women to test the fetus (pre-natal screening); (iii) on *in vitro* embryos before they are inserted into a woman's womb (pre-implantation screening); (iv) on children and adults to test for some genetic condition or for so-called 'hypersusceptability' to contracting a particular condition.

Germ line   The series of cells in the body that eventually develop into egg and sperm cells (**gametes**, also called germ cells).

GIFT: Gamete Intrafallopian Transfer   A variation of IVF in which collected eggs and sperm are injected into the woman's fallopian tube so that fertilisation can take place there, instead of in the laboratory dish.

in vitro **fertilisation: IVF** Joining of egg and sperm outside the female body and in a laboratory dish. It necessitates using other laboratory and medical procedures on women, such as **superovulation, ultrasound, laparoscopic egg retrival,** and **embryo transfer.**

Laparoscopy Visual examination of ovaries (or other abdominal organs) by insertion of a light guide through a small incision in the woman's abdominal wall. Eggs can be removed during laparoscopy, by the insertion of a suction device and a forceps for grasping the woman's ovary. As an egg retrieval method it requires anaesthesia and distention of the abdomen with a carbon dioxide gas mixture.

Lavage see **Embryo flushing**

Menstrual regulation or **menstrual extraction** A suction method of extracting the uterine lining which is built up during the menstrual cycle. It is carried out within fourteen days of the missed menstrual period. It can be used as an early abortion method if a woman thinks she may be pregnant. It is easily performed, without anaesthesia, and takes only a few minutes.

Molecular biology The study of the structure and function of large molecules associated with living organisms, especially DNA and proteins.

Molecule A term used in chemistry and biochemistry to describe a basic unit of matter. All matter is composed of elements (or atoms) such as hydrogen, oxygen and carbon. Elements combine to form molecules. For example, when two hydrogen atoms chemically combine with one oxygen atom the result is a molecule of water (H_2O). The 'molecules of life' (e.g. DNA and proteins) are much larger and more complex.

Nucleus substitution A cloning method in mammals. The nucleus is removed from an unfertilised egg cell and replaced with a new nucleus taken from a body cell (see **chromosome** and **gamete**). The egg may then develop as if it were fertilised. Also called **nuclear transplantation.**

Oocyte (egg cell) see **Gamete**

Parthenogenesis Development of an organism from an unfertilised egg. It occurs naturally in many plants and a few animals. Scientists have induced mouse eggs to undergo parthanogenetic cell devision for a brief time, and an IVF team in Australia observed brief parthenogenesis in women's eggs.

Pelvic inflammatory disease (PID) In women, any infection and inflammation of the pelvic organs which is caused by bacteria or viruses.

The infection often localises in the fallopian tubes. PIDs are a cause of fertility problems.

Progesterone   A hormone produced in the ovaries after ovulation, and by the placenta during pregnancy. Synthetic progesterones were first developed for use as contraceptives. They work by interfering with the processes necessary for ovulation, egg movement, development of the uterine lining, and cervical mucus production. They have immediate adverse effects, such as irregular bleeding. Little is know of the long-term effects, and risks may include loss of fertility and alterations in the woman's immunological system. As drugs they are also prescribed to treat premenstrual tension and for women with fertility problems, for example to prevent miscarriage.

Sex selection   A term which refers to either (i) the identification of the sex of an already existing embryo (e.g. during **amniocentesis, CVS,** or pre-implantation screening of an *in vitro* embryo); or (ii) the engineering of the sex of an embryo before fertilisation occurs, more accurately called sex pre-selection.

Sterilisation   A surgical procedure whose purpose is to render a person unable to reproduce. The most common type of sterilisation for women today is tubal ligation, tying off the fallopian tubes. Other types are hysterectomy (removal of the uterus) and oopherectomy (removal of the ovaries). **Sterilisation abuse** refers to efforts to pressure or coerce women to undergo sterilisation without informed consent.

Superovulation   A woman is administered a regimen of fertility drugs and hormones to induce the maturation and release of more than one egg at a single menstrual cycle so that several eggs can be collected. The eggs can then be used to make embryos, for 'egg donation', for egg or embryo freezing, for experimentation, or for other procedures such as GIFT and TUDOR. The risks to the woman from the use of superovulatory drugs include hyperstimulation of the ovaries and the formation of cysts, both of which can be serious conditions and can adversely effect a woman's fertility. The long-term risks of superovulation regimens has never been investigated, but some of the drugs used are related to known carcinogens.

'Surrogate' mother   A woman who becomes pregnant and carries a child for another person or couple. She may provide the egg and be inseminated, or she may receive an IVF embryo if another woman's egg is used. The term 'surrogate' is incorrect, as the woman who bears the child is a real mother, not a substitute mother.

TUDOR: Transvaginal Ultrasound Directed Oocyte Recovery   A method of egg collection introduced as an alternative to laparoscopic egg recovery. The woman's bladder is emptied and filled with saline solution. A needle for pulling out the eggs is inserted through her vagina and into the bladder

and towards the ovary. Ultrasound scanning guides the doctor moving the needle. Eggs are more difficult to grasp than in **laparoscopy**, and damage to the bladder is a risk.

Ultrasound scanning The use of high frequency sound waves to show visual outlines of internal body structures. The picture (or scan) is shown on a television screen. In obstetrics it has been used since the 1960s to visualise the fetus inside the woman's womb to determine fetal growth and gestational age, and to look for 'abnormalities' or 'disorders' of the uterus, placenta and fetus. Ultrasound can be used to detect the sex of the fetus. It also enables a doctor to carry out other obstetrical interventions on the pregnant woman, such as amniocentesis. In IVF practice, vaginal ultrasound is used to monitor the woman's ovulation and as part of egg recovery (see **TUDOR**). Ultrasound is now widely used on pregnant women for antenatal diagnosis, although no long-term studies on its effects have as yet been reported. Also called ultrasonography and sonogram.

Notes

Chapter 1: Setting the ethic

1. See the Ethics Advisory Board (1979) of the US Department of Health Education and Welfare for a summary of the first wave of the ethical debates in the scientific literature over IVF issues.

In this book I do not go into the vast literature by professional ethicists and bioethicists who have been addressing the new reproductive technologies. A great deal appears in the medical and scientific literature (see References), and in the *Hastings Centre Report* (US) and the *Journal of Medical Ethics*, the journal of the British Institute of Medical Ethics. Anne Donchin reviews some of the views in the mainstream ethics debate in her article 'The Future of Mothering: Technology and Feminist Theory' (1986) in *Hypatia: A Journal of Feminist Philosophy* 1, 2, pp. 121–39.

2. IVF practitioners require ripe eggs, that is eggs at a certain stage in development. This means that they must extract eggs from women at a particular time: as the eggs are maturing, but before they are released from the ovaries. In the past, when experimenters tried to use 'immature' eggs, the IVF procedure failed. This was a limiting factor, and so researchers are working on maturing women's unripe eggs in the laboratory. This project is, for example, being carried out at Edwards and Steptoe's Bourn Hall Clinic in Cambridge, England.

3. By ideology I mean the representations and images which function within a given society at a specific time, and which are related to the views and norms which play a part in structuring that society.

4. I took this quote from a superb article by Jalna Hanmer, 'Locating Women in Reproductive and Genetic Engineering', 1986, pp. 6–21. The quote comes from *Journal of the American Medical Association*, 1972, Genetic Engineering: Reprieve, 220, 10, pp. 1355, 57. It is cited in *Genetic Engineering: Evolution of a Technological Issue*, 1972, US House of Representatives, 92nd Congress.

5. From a group discussion at the Women's Reproductive Rights Information Centre, London, 16 March 1987.

6. Professor Jerome Strauss made the statement, that IVF has altered the practice of obstetrics and gynaecology, during a discussion with me on 31 December 1985.

7.   Short's remarks appear in the report of the Ethics Advisory Board (1979), which quotes the paper he prepared for the Board, in Chapter III, nt. 27.

8.   IVF advocates certainly understand the moral paradox of allowing some people (IVF practitioners and research scientists) to handle embryos while the abortion laws restrict women's reproductive self-determination in the name of the protection of embryos. For an obvious example, I wrote a short article outlining this point in the University of York News Sheet, in 1986, in response to an article by Dr Henry Leese, who was carrying out a human embryo research project there in collaboration with Robert Edwards. A year later, Dr Leese presented a *public* lecture, open to the community, on the social implications of IVF. He never mentioned this particular moral paradox which I and other women in York have been voicing. Instead, the ethical discussion on IVF which he presented covered the same basic points which IVF advocates had been arguing since the 1970s, as if no new insights were relevent. (The articles were 'Research on Human Embryos', by Henry Leese, University of York News Sheet, Issue 186, Jan.–Feb. 1986; and 'Embryo Research: A Woman's Point of View', by Patricia Spallone, University of York News Sheet, Issue 187, March 1986. Dr Leese's public lecture was 'Human In Vitro Fertilisation: A Case Study In Science and Its Social Implications', delivered 19 May 1987, at the University of York, as part of the Open Course series.)

Another example of living with the moral paradox is the IVF situation in the Republic of Ireland. An amendment to the Irish constitution passed in 1983 guarantees the embryo's right to full human status, and so human embryo research is not allowed there. However, IVF as a clinical treatment is being offered, while researchers in other countries do the preliminary work of experimentation on embryos considered a crime in Ireland.

9.   As I will show in Chapters 4 and 8, IVF is being used to normalise a certain kind of family, the nuclear family, defined as patrilineal, of two generations, comprising a heterosexual couple living together with their children. Historically the nuclear family is the male-headed household, whose rules and regulations place women in economic and social dependence on men, supported in law and by the institutions and norms which structure Western societies. When the question of adverse consequences to the 'family' was introduced by ethicists, IVF advocates in Britain, the USA and Australia argued that their application affirmed family values within heterosexual marriage, and even more, that IVF saves marriages suffering for lack of children.

10.   'Informed consent' is problematic for patient-subjects. Most therapies are established within a narrow medical science context, and most new therapies are used on the basis of professional consensus without evidence of their efficacy and dangers. Also, they are offered to people as a 'choice' with little appreciation for the fact that practitioners and hospitals approve certain therapies and thereby preclude alternative approaches. See Hubbard (1982).

11.   I owe thanks to Janice Raymond for giving me the words to express my perspective. In *A Passion for Friends* (1986), she coins the word

'*heteroreality*, the world view that women exist always in relation to man, has consistently perceived women together as women alone' (p. 3).

Chapter 2: The status of the embryo

1. Western thought and culture about the 'value of embryonic life' from the time of the Greeks to the present day is a revealing history of ideology-in-the-making. I cannot go into that history here but two sources that cover part of it are *The Death of Nature* (1982) by Carolyn Merchant and *Reproductive Rituals* (1984) by Angus McLaren. Merchant shows that throughout that history women were consistently perceived as passive beings of generation; even in 'alternative', seemingly egalitarian theories of procreation, the female's role was still considered 'less perfect' than the male's role. McLaren looks at the relationship between medical, legal and Church views about pregnancy and the beliefs and practices of ordinary people in England before the Enlightenment.

The classic example of nature-from-the-male-viewpoint is the 'discovery' by Anton von Leeuwenhoek which launched a new preformation theory in embryology. Preformationists believed that an entire human being was present in the 'seed' (sperm or egg), and needed only to grow without the addition of any new parts. Using the latest in late seventeenth-century technology, the microscope, Leeuwenhoek claimed to have seen a tiny preformed person within the sperm cell.

Although preformation theories sound silly today, we have a contemporary version of it in the idea that all the information necessary to make a human being exists in the genes in the fertilised egg. This interpretation is not as far-fetched as one might think. 'Genetic identity' of the IVF embryo and 'genetic relationship' is of central concern to ethicists, medical scientists, and government committees discussing the NRTs. The philosopher Mary Warnock, who chaired the British Warnock Committee into IVF issues, explained in an interview that they decided on a fourteen day upper limit for 'human embryo' research on the basis of the embryos 'genetic identity'. She believes, 'the genetic composition of the resulting child is not determined for 14 days' (Dunn, 1984), and thought this criterion was more important for deciding when to protect the embryo than the question of whether an embryo is alive or not.

2. I had an informal conversation with IVF practitioner Simon B. Fishel, on 8 September 1987, in Birmingham, after we both took part in a television programme about infertility (Central ITV's 'The Time . . . The Place'). To rebut my contention that the road to IVF necessitates experimentation on women, Dr Fishel said that preliminary knowledge was gained from animals. He then stated that women were biologically no different from sheep, but added, we are emotionally different. This view splits women in two, a gendered human being and a sexed biological animal. As I discuss in Chapter 5, it obscures the fact that women are the subject of the reproductive scientists' experiments. Also, I should add, IVF practice was not firmly established on animals before it was used on women (see Chapter 5).

3. At a meeting of the York Women's Reproductive Rights Campaign in 1987, one member who works in a local hospital related to us that many pregnant women find ultrasound scanning an upsetting experience. Rather than finding the picture of the fetus comforting, they find it disconcerting. Many feel they have not been given adequate information about what kind of image to expect. An article which touches on this is 'Ultrasound in Pregnancy: Should it be Routine?' in the *Drug and Therapeutics Bulletin* (1985).

4. This information comes from conversations with two BPAS personnel in September 1987. I owe thanks to Marilyn Crawshaw for pointing out that legal restrictions on abortion translate to even greater restrictions on women than the letter of the law allows, during a conversation on 7 September 1987. (Women in Britain were being threatened by yet another private member's bill aiming to restrict the upper time limit for abortion to eighteen weeks. As I complete the proofs of this book David Alton's anti-abortion bill failed.)

5. The British Medical Association was tentative in its support of the RCOG *et al.* Report (1985) recommending further restriction of the Abortion Act 1967, although they were represented on the committee that drew up the report (Timmins, 1985).

6. The fourteen day limit first appeared as an official government recommendation in the report of the US's Ethics Advisory Board (EAB) hearings (1979). The Warnock Report (1984) does not refer to the EAB recommendation. Following the Warnock Report, many other Western countries adopted the fourteen day limit.

7. The Council for Science and Society (CSS) working party to investigate IVF and related issues, including artificial insemination and surrogacy, also included Walter Bodmer, a world renowned human geneticist. The chair, Rev. Gordon Dunstan is an IVF advocate (Dunstan, 1983). Their report was published a few weeks before the British Government inquiry, the Warnock Report. The CSS working party 'reflects the views and interests of the members of the Warnock Committee' (Veitch, 1984b).

8. During a discussion in Oxford on 15 February 1987, Anne McLaren related this story to me about the coining of the word pre-embryo by a lay member of the VLA.

    I chronicled the evolution of the term 'pre-embryo' with the help of the following references: Clarke, 1985b; Huxley, 1985; Turney, 1985; Ironside, 1985; Clarke, 1986; Davies, 1986; McLaren, 1986a; McLaren, 1986b; Connor, 1985; *Ob Gyn News*, 1985a; Morgan, 1987; American Fertility Society Ethics Committee, 1986, pp. vii and 285; MRC/RCOG Voluntary Licensing Authority, 1985 and 1986; *Nature*, 1987.

9. Many people are unaware that mid-term fetuses acquired from abortions have been used for scientific research. See Austin, 1973 and McCance, 1977 for examples and a scientist's review of the early history.

Chapter 3: IVF on women

1. I used many primary sources (published material and statements by

IVF practitioners) in painting this profile of a basic IVF procedure. Among them are the following representative articles from IVF laboratories in Britain, Australia, the USA and Denmark: Edwards, 1965; Edwards *et al.*, 1966; Edwards *et al.*, 1969; Steptoe and Edwards, 1970; Edwards, Steptoe and Purdy, 1970; Edwards and Steptoe, 1983; Fleming *et al.*, 1985; Forman *et al.*, 1985; Jacobs *et al.*, 1985; Johnston *et al.*, 1981; Lindenberg *et al.*, 1985; Lopata, 1980; Marrs, 1984; Marrs *et al.*, 1984; Pittaway, 1984; Sandow, 1983; Sher *et al.*, 1984; Trounson and Conti, 1982; Trounson *et al.*, 1983a; Wood *et al.*, 1984; Yovich *et al.*, 1982; Yovich *et al.*, 1983. Feminist works which helped me in formulating this chapter are cited within the text. Also, see Greenfeld and Haseltine (1986).

2. For a comprehensive, demystified description of the known hormonal events of reproduction, and some of the drugs used for fertility therapy, see Regina Pfeiffer and Katherine Whitlock's *Fertility Awareness* (1984).

Chapter 4: The domain of medicine

1. Ultrasound technology has its roots in warfare; it was developed as a submarine detection method in the First World War. The National Institutes of Health in the USA concluded in 1984 that routine diagnostic ultrasound scanning during pregnancy could not be justified by known evidence; but in Britain an RCOG working party concluded that routine ultrasound at sixteen to eighteen weeks was justifiable (Neilson, 1986).

In Britain, social scientist Ann Oakley (1986) looked critically at the history of ultrasonography in obstetrics. Among her many illuminating points, she showed that the dangers of ultrasound have not yet been adequately evaluated, and further, that the use of techniques such as ultrasound displace a woman's subjective knowledge of her pregnancy for what doctors believe is the 'objective' data of the machine, thus transforming the social relationships of those who use them. Also see Cross, 1986; Hubbard, 1984; and *Drug and Therapeutics Bulletin*, 1985.

2. Most women's reproductive organs include two fallopian tubes which link the two ovaries to the womb. During a woman's menstrual cycle, an egg is released from one of the ovaries and travels up the fallopian tube on its way to the womb; fertilisation of egg and sperm usually takes place in the fallopian tube. If the tubes are inflamed or blocked, it could result in inability to conceive.

3. The data and statistics in this section come from the following medical sources. Reports on the link between the IUD and infertility appear in *British Medical Journal*, 1978 and Anderson, 1985. Relevant medical textbooks are Garcia *et al.* (eds), 1984; Huggins, 1984; Wallach and Kempers (eds), 1979. The relevant World Health Organisation reports are Diczfalusy, 1986; Wagatsuma, 1981; WHO Fourteenth Annual Report, 1985. Information about *chlamydia trachomatis* infections and fertility problems is in Ridgeway *et al.*, 1983; Rowland *et al.*, 1985; Rowland and Moss, 1985; Moss and Hawkswell, 1986.

I owe thanks to all the workers at the Women's Reproductive Rights Information Centre in London, whose information was also a help in compiling this section. For published information on known causes of infertility and on the various therapies from a feminist perspective see Pfeiffer and Whitlock, 1984 and Pfeffer and Woollett, 1983.

4. A 'treatment cycle' entails the steps in IVF from superovulation to embryo insertion; if a woman does not get pregnant during a treatment cycle, she may go through the entire procedure again. When IVF teams use frozen embryos, the procedures are modified.

5. I thank Christine Crowe for her suggestion that I expand on the point about the use of the word 'mother' by IVF practitioners and for pointing out the quote from Adrienne Rich. See Crowe's article, 'The Reproductive Fix' (1985).

6. The obstetrician, I later learned from a London midwife, was Ian Craft, who became the director of an IVF programme at the Cromwell Hospital in London. In 1987, Craft was berated by the Voluntary Licensing Authority for refusing to adhere to the VLA guidelines on the maximum numbers of *in vitro* embryos to be inserted in a woman's womb (see Chapter 3).

Chapter 5: The status of scientific knowledge

1. This view of nature as exploitable is not monolithic, but exists in parallel with a seemingly contradictary view, where nature is an 'ideal'. It is not uncommon for those who use animals in exploitative situations to also be conservationists. All ecologists are not asking for a radical change in how industries, governments and science treat nature. One such view is exemplified by the editorials in the British magazine for the privileged, *Country Life*; their message is to conserve nature for its aesthetic pleasures. Yet the readership includes those who make their living from and support environmentally hazardous industries. For another example, the more scientifically minded ecologist might argue conservation to maintain 'genetic diversity'. This is not the place to discuss these parallel views, but I wish to point out that underlying the dominating capitalist and patriarchal world view, nature serves Man [sic] economically, intellectually, aesthically.

2. During a conversation with me on 8 September 1987, in Birmingham, IVF practitioner Simon Fishel stated that the first evidence of fertilisation of a woman's egg with a man's sperm was documented in a photograph published in 1948 by Menkin and Rock. However, historical surveys of IVF on women by the US Ethics Advisory Board (1979) and by Robert Edwards (1983a) declare that there was no demonstrable evidence of egg division/fertilisation *in vitro* until the 1960s. My concern, though, is not with who deserves the dubious credit for the first demonstrable fertilisation of a woman's egg in a laboratory, but rather the fact that women's bodies were being used for these experiments for decades.

3. *A Matter of Life* by Edwards and Steptoe is an effusive

self-congratulatory portrait of themselves, a revelation of their intentions and goals, and their self-perceptions. I found it a stark contrast to the portrait of these same men made in *Our Miracle Called Louise*, the story told by parents of the first baby born by IVF, Lesley and John Brown.

4. All these arguments, for example, appeared in editorials in the journal *Nature*, see Chapter 1 and the articles under *Nature* (as author) in the References.

5. A great deal has been written on the social and cultural aspects of technologies. Among them, Joan Rothschild (ed.) (1983) *Machina Ex Dea: Feminist Perspectives on Technology*, Pergamon, New York; Brighton Women and Science Group (1980) *Alice Through the Microscope*, Virago, London; Pamela D'Onofrio and Sheila Pfafflin (eds) (1982) *Scientific–Technological Change and the Role of Women in Development*, UN Institute for Training and Research, Westview Press. Boulder; Hilary Rose and Steven Rose (eds) (1976) *The Political Economy of Science* and *The Radicalization of Science*, Macmillan, London; Arnold Pacey (1983) *The Culture of Technology*, Basic Blackwell, Oxford.

6. 'When Nature Fails' is the title of a video prepared by the pharmaceutical company Organon to be shown to prospective IVF clients (Burfoot, 1987).

7. Many women are writing about the social pressures placed on women due to technology. See Arditti *et al.*, 1984; Crowe, 1987a; Rothman, 1986.

8. Robert Edwards evaluated social, legal and moral issues of IVF as early as 1974 in the *Quarterly Review of Biology*. For a general example, 'The Royal Society and the Genesis of the Scientific Advisory Committee to Britain's War Cabinet, 1939–1940' by William McGucken is a revealing account of one successful effort of the scientific élite in Britain of engineering their way into the halls of political power against the objections of government officials (*Notes and Records of the Royal Society* 1978–9, 33, pp. 87–116).

Chapter 6: The new genetics

1. For the history of scientific appreciation of Mendel's work see Kelves, (1985, pp. 43–5) and Peters (1959).

2. DNA is a helical-shaped molecule composed of two chains of nucleotides wound around each other and linked by chemical bonds. Genes, special pieces of DNA, 'code' for proteins; that is, the sequence of nucleotides along the gene carries information for the production in the cell of a specific protein.

3. The DNA fingerprinting scheme is also racist. It would not apply to White people immigrating from Commonwealth countries, but primarily to immigrants from the Indian subcontinent, as a spokewoman for the Welfare of Immigrants stressed (Travis, 1986).

4. Many known inherited disorders are associated with a specific ethnic population. These associations have in the past and present been used

against certain groups of people. The historian Daniel Kevles chronicles some of the racist practices of eugenists in the USA in his book *In the Name of Eugenics* (1985). Paula Bradish (1987) exposd a blatent present-day example in West Germany, in which a geneticist cited the inability to digest milk (lactose intolerance) as an example of a genetic 'defect'. As Bradish points out, this condition is common in the peoples of Asia and Africa, who perhaps do not perceive it as a 'defect' since milk is not a part of the normal diet of adults in these regions of the world.

The direction of genetic research on human populations has taken place in the context of racist, as well as sexist, Western ideas. Genetic principles were and are used to explain both gender and racial differences, and to support racist and sexist practices with scientific 'fact'.

5.   Many women have written about their own and other women's experiences with genetic screening. See Rakusen, 1982; Rapp, 1984; Saxton, 1984; Rothman, 1986. Three feminist collections with articles analysing genetic screening, disabled rights, and eugenics are *Test-tube Women* (1984) by Artditti *et al.* (eds); *Man-Made Women* by Corea *et al.* (1985); and *Made to Order* (1987) by Spallone and Steinberg (eds).

6.   New capabilities in gene analysis take genetic screening beyond reproduction. Researchers have identified genes in some individuals which supposedly make us more 'susceptible' to certain illnesses. 'Hypersensitivity' to asbestos is one such genetically related condition. Some people, because of our genes, are more likely to get lung cancer from breathing asbestos fibres. Employers in several countries have shown interest in screening all job applicants and workers for the new range of genetically related 'conditions' and 'susceptabilities'; such tests, they believe, would be useful in deciding who is genetically 'fit' to work. This is yet another example of defining the cause of the problem on an individual's genes, not the polluted environment or hazardous working conditions.

7.   Since the early 1980s political activists in the USA, Britain, and West Germany have fought to prevent the release of genetically engineered bacteria, viruses and plants into the environment. In 1987, in the USA, the biotechnology company Advanced Genetic Sciences was given permission by the government to release genetically engineered bacteria created to protect strawberry plants from frost. That same year, the US Patent Office decided to permit the patenting of organisms that have been genetically altered by scientists through genetic engineering. Activist Jeremy Rifkin condemned the decision saying, 'They're saying that there is no difference between living things and electric toasters' (Joyce, 1987). See Linda Bullard's article, 'Killing Us Softly: Toward a Feminist Analysis of Genetic Engineering' (1987).

8.   An enormous amount of money and resources from public and private sectors is pumped into biotechnology research and development. See The International Biotechnology Directory 1985 by J. Coombs (Macmillan) for a breakdown of funding, organisations and activities.

9.   I am referring to the marketing of infant formula, dried milk manufactured by certain food multinationals to be used in place of women's breast milk. In poor countries, the use of dried milk for baby food was

responsible for the deaths of millions of babies. Pressure groups arose to restrict the marketing campaign of multinationals, who tried to deny that the product was dangerous for use in these countries. The scandal provoked an international boycott against the Nestlé corporation, the world leader in infant formula, in the early 1980s. For details of the events and the campaign against Nestlé see Andrew Chetley's *The Politics of Baby Foods* (1986).

Chapter 7: The new eugenics

1.   A look at the topics and speakers during the annual symposia of the Eugenics Society in London reflects that eugenists of various professions consider all these topics of eugenic interest.

2.   Robyn Rowland cites many references in which IVF practitioners make eugenic claims of superior health and social adjustment of IVF babies. See Rowland, 1985, p. 539.

3.   Malthus' theory states that population increases in a geometrical ratio and subsistance (food) only in an arithmetical ratio. He argued that population is necessarily limited by the 'checks' of vice and misery. He later amended his opinion on 'checks'. He was made a member of the Royal Society in 1819. Charles Darwin said Malthus' principle inspired him.

4.   I do not mean to give the impression that the authors of *The Humanist Frame* were purposely trying to modernise Galton's theories, They did not acknowledge their link with his work. I am making the link here.

5.   Within the scientific community since the 1960s, there have been ongoing debates over 'biological determinism', the relationship between genetic endowment and behaviour. To put it simply, on one side are the more sociobiology minded arguing that human traits and behaviour are for a large part genetically determined. Their antagonists are scientists who reject the primacy of the gene principle for a more 'holistic' approach, where environmental and social factors which effect human behaviour are better recognised. However, many of the 'good guys' who debunk genetic determinism do not reject the genetic thesis that there is a genetic basis of behaviour or human traits. I do not have space to go into my criticism here, but one article which illustrates the point in the context of the IQ/race controversy in the USA is Bodmer and Cavalli-Sforza (1970). They vehemently rejected Jensen's scientific 'proof' that Blacks were inherently less intelligent than Whites, but they still believed that intelligence is 'probably influenced by the combined action of many genes' (p. 19). For a feminist critique of sociobiology see Bleier (1984).

6.   The editors of *Nature* enjoy positions of authority in the IVF debate. David Davies, a former editor, sat on the Warnock Committee which made recommendations to the British Government on IVF issues. Editor John Maddox sat on a committee of scientists and politicians formed in the early 1970s by the British Association for the Advancement of Science to address the ethical issues arising from advances in biology, including artificial reproduction techniques.

7.   Many women have written critically on the birth control movement, and its links with eugenics and population control. See for example *Alice Through the Microscope* (1980) by the Brighton Women and Science Group and *Women's Body, Women's Right* by Linda Gordon (1976).

8.   Contrary to the dominant Western myths about 'Third World' dependency are the facts that foreign food 'aid' is not channelled to the hungry and impoverished, and that a country such as Bangladesh possesses the natural resources to feed itself. See *Needless Hunger: Voices from a Bangladesh Village* (1979) by Betsy Hartmann and James K. Boyce published by the Institute for Food and Development Policy in San Francisco.

There is a growing body of literature on women and development, much which considers international and national population control policies. Betsy Hartman's (1987) 'A Womb of One's Own: The Real Population Problem', discusses some of the issues involved.

9.   I have kept the discussion of eugenics centred on the activities of industrialised Western countries, plus their impact on 'Third World' countries. I wish to add that Japanese women activists are resisting the eugenic practices and policies of the Japanese state. They make quite clear that the state's desire to control population quantity and quality is caught up in their perception of the population as an economic and military resource. They see the eugenic ideal in the context of a desirable young labour force in an aging society, and they make important links between the state's desire to keep women's reproduction in the context of marriage and the prohibition of women's rights to abortion (for anything but negative eugenic reasons). This information comes from published and unpublished documents circulated at the international Emergency Conference on the New Reproductive Technologies in 1985 in Vällinge.

Chapter 8: A matter of state interest

1.   Comment during the European Women's Conference on Reproduction Technology and Genetic Engineering, 1986, Palma.

2.   Jenny Teichman's *Illegitimacy* (1982) includes interesting discussions on the way governments in different countries have 'reformed' the concept of illegitimacy to maintain men's rights over women's reproduction.

A recent example comes from Maria Jose Varela, Secretary of the Commission of Women Lawyers of the College of Lawyers of Cataluna, in her 'Critical Analysis of the Spanish Parliamentary Commission's Report on the Study of Human IVF and AI', presented 11 October 1986 at the Women's European Conference on Reproductive Technology and Genetic Engineering in Palma. She explained that although Spain abolished the legal distinction between legitimacy and illegitimacy, the distinction persists. Government recommendations on IVF and AID reflect the fact that Spanish law still recognises the Napoleonic code which upholds the rights of the husband as the legal father of any child his wife bears, even a

child who is known to have been conceived with another man's sperm (as in AID). Not surprisingly, under Spanish law a natural mother may still be challenged to prove her maternal 'fitness' by husband and the state.
3. The Victoria Waller Committee was not so sure about strict anonymity. They feel a less secretive approach will prove preferable for the child, both psychologically and for better medical records and follow-up studies. They also recognise a child's 'right to know' her or his genetic parents.

Chapter 9: Transforming reality

1. As I mentioned in Chapter 4, Ann Oakley's (1986) article on ultrasound scanning shows quite clearly the intangible dangers of ultrasound; women's subjective knowledge of pregnancy is being displaced by the quite different 'objective' data doctors glean from ultrasound machines.
2. This quote comes from an unpublished paper in the documentation of the Emergency Conference on the New Reproductive Technologies in 1985. Write to Committee Against Revision of Eugenic Protection Law, c/o JOKI, NAKAZAWA Build. 3F, Araki-cho 23, Shinjuku-ku, Tokyo, Japan.
3. The quoted phrases and C. P. Snow's comments come from Ronald Clark's *The Greatest Power on Earth: The Story of Nuclear Fission* (1980). Also see *The Energy Question* (1976) by Gerald Foley with Charlotte Nassim. A passage which they quote from nuclear pioneer Frederick Soddy's *Matter and Energy* (1912) succinctly reveals the scientific perception about the social and economic impact of the twentieth-century discoveries in nuclear physics.
Another significant historical parallel is the advice of Viennese physicist Erwin Schrödinger to biologists in *What is Life* (1944). He suggested that nature's fundamental laws of life could be found in the gene within the cell, just as physicists had found the fundamental laws of physical matter inside the atom.
4. FINRRAGE began in 1984 at an interrational women's conference in Gröningen, The Netherlands. The founding members talk about its beginnings in a preface to *Made to Order: The Myth of Reproductive and Genetic Progress* (1987) edited by Patricia Spallone and Deborah Lynn Steinberg. Also see 'International Report' in the same collection.
5. In the April 1987 issue of the US feminist magazine *MS* there was a letter from a women who said that after years of being unable to become pregnant, she finally did so by placing egg whites in her vagina. She read in *MS* that this method was used successfully by some women who had problems conceiving. She and her partner had gone through five years of fertility tests, but there were no obvious problems ('unexplained' infertility). She theorised that the sperm needed a bit of pull, which the egg white provided.
6. Alison Solomon's presentation at the Dublin conference is

unpublished, but an article based on it is due to appear in *The Exploitation of Infertility: Women and Reproductive Technologies* (Women's Press, 1989) edited by Renate Klein. This book is devoted to the experiences of women with fertility problems, how infertility affected their lives, and their experiences with IVF and related procedures. Or see Solomon's (1988) 'Integrating Infertility Crisis Counselling into Feminist Practice', *Journal of Reproductive and Genetic Engineering: International Feminist Analysis*, vol. 1, no. 1.

Published sources

The list of references to this book is not a comprehensive bibliography, nor does it include many of the books and articles which informed my thinking about reproductive and genetic technology. The published material on the subject is huge. And the feminist and mainstream works on related issues, such as sexuality, kinship, and women in development, is also enormous. In this section I wish to organise some of the sources which appear in the References, and add some information. For the few sources below which do not appear in the references, full information is given.

(a) Feminist works

The growing literature on feminist criticisms of the new reproductive technologies includes Gena Corea's *The Mother Machine* (1985), the anthologies *Test-Tube Women* (1984) edited by Rita Arditti, Renate Duelli Klein and Shelley Minden; *Man-Made Women* (1985) by Gena Corea *et al.*; *Made to Order* (1987) edited by Patricia Spallone and Deborah Lynn Steinberg. On birthing technology there is Jill Rakusen and Nick Davidson's *Out of Our Hands* (1982); and Barabara Katz Rothman's *The Tentative Pregnancy* (1986).

Also see articles by Farida Akhter 'Contraceptive Technology and the Coercive Reorganization of Society' (1986a) and 'Depopulating Bangladesh' (1986b); Rita Arditti's ' "Surrogate Mothering" Exploits Women' (1987); Christine Crowe's 'The Reproductive Fix' (1985); articles by Jalna Hanmer 'Sex Predetermination, Artificial Insemination and the Maintenance of Male-dominated Culture' (1981) and 'Locating Women in Reproductive and Genetic Engineering' (1986); Ellen Hopkins' 'High Tech Pregnancies' (1985); Ruth Hubbard's 'Prenatal Diagnosis and Eugenic Ideology' (1985); Sheila Kitzenger's 'Battle of Birth Rights' (1985); Lena Koch and Janice Morgall's 'Toward a Feminist Assessment of Reproductive Technology' (1987); Françoise Laborie's 'New Reproductive Technologies: News From France' (1988); Maria Mies' 'The Social Origins of the Sexual Division of Labour' (1981); Ann Oakley's 'The History of Ultrasonography in Obstetrics' (1986); Robyn Rowland's 'A Child At Any Price?' (1985); Patricia Spallone's 'The Warnock Report' (1985). In German is *Frauen Gegen Gentechnik und Reproduktionstechnik* (Women

216

Against Gene Technology and Reproductive Technology) which is the documentation from the Bonn conference in April, 1985. Forthcoming is *The Exploitation of infertility: Women and Reproductive Technologies edited by Renate Klein (Women's Press)*.

Related feminist works are Mary O'Brien's *The Politics of Reproduction* (1981); Gena Corea's *The Hidden Malpractice* (1985), Harper & Row, New York; Mary Daly's *Gyn/ecology* (1979); Barbara Ehrenrich and Deirdre English's *For Her Own Good* (1979); Linda Gordon's *Women's Body, Women's Right* (1976); Ruth Bleier's *Science and Gender* (1984); Sandra Harding's *The Science Question in Feminism* (1986); The Association of Radical Midwives' 'The Vision' (1986); Rosalie Bertell's *No Immediate Danger* (1985); Andrea Dworkin's *Right Wing Women* (1983); Anna Davin's article 'Imperialism and Motherhood' (1978); Maria Mies' *Patriarchy and Accumulation on a World Scale* (1986); Naomi Pfeffer and Anne Woollett's *The Experience of Infertility* (1983); Adrienne Rich's *Of Women Born* (1976); Anja Meulenblatt *et al.* (eds), *A Creative Tension* (1984); Jenny Teichman's *Illegitimacy* (1982). Women's health movement books include Regina Asaph Pfeiffer and Katherine Whitlock's *Fertility Awareness* (1984) and the Boston Women's Health Book Collective's *The New Our Bodies Ourselves* (1985), Simon & Schuster, New York.

A selected bibliography on the social, economic and political implications of the NRTs and the feminist critique of science, compiled by Sarah Franklin, can be found in *Made to Order* (1987) edited by Patricia Spallone and Deborah Lynn Steinberg. It lists many other feminist and non-feminist sources. A list of resources and further reading also appears in *Test-tube Women* (1985) edited by Rita Arditti, Renate Duelli Klein and Shelley Minden.

Also see *Journal of Reproductive and Genetic Engineering: International Feminist Analysis*, whose first issue appeared in spring 1988.

Other criticisms of the new biotechnologies which in several areas overlap feminist criticisms are Gordon Rattray Taylor, 1968 and Jeremy Rifkin, 1985. Essential information is provided in Maurice Pappworth, 1967, on past experimentation on women and men in clinical medicine; and John Elkington, 1986 on reproductive toxicology and the effects on health of offspring.

(b) Issues by chapter

In several notes throughout the book I list further reading on certain topics. I will not repeat the sources here, but only direct the reader to them.

Chapter 1, note 1 mentions sources on the first and second waves of the professional ethics debates on the NRTs, and sources on medical ethics. Also see the series of books *Genetics and the Law* (volumes I, II, III) edited by Aubrey Milunsky and George J. Annas.

Two important books that cover the history of embryo-centred views in Western thought about reproduction are listed in Chapter 2, note 1; also see J. Needham (1959) *A History of Embryology*, Cambridge University

Press and T. J. Horder *et al*. (eds) (1986) *A History of Embryology: British Society for Developmental Biology*, Symposium 8.

Within Chapter 2 are several references to mainstream and feminist literature on the use of 'fetal rights' and its relationship to medical ideas and practice. In addition, two extremely useful, detailed articles on the situation in the USA are Dawn E. Johnsen (1986) 'The Creation of Fetal Rights: Conflicts with Women's Constitutional Rights to Liberty, Privacy, and Equal Protection', *The Yale Law Journal*, vol. 95, pp. 599–625; and Nancy K. Rhoden (1987) 'The Judge in the Delivery Room: The Emergence of Court-Ordered Caesareans', *California Law Review*, vol. 74, pp. 1951–2030.

The evolution of the term 'pre-embryo' can be chronicled from references given in Chapter 2, note 8.

Two scientific sources on experimentation on human fetuses acquired from abortions are in Chapter 2, note 9.

I used many books and articles from the medical/scientific literature. Chapter 3, note 1 lists those reporting the use of IVF on women for clinical practice. Also see the general science journals *Nature, Science, The New Scientist, The Proceedings of the Royal Society, Quarterly Review of Biology*; and the medical journals *The British Medical Journal, The Lancet, The American Journal of Obstetrics and Gynaecology, Journal of the American Medical Association, The New England Journal of Medicine, Fertility and Sterility, Ob Gyn News, The Journal of Medical Ethics. The Journal of In Vitro Fertilisation and Embryo Transfer* appeared in 1984, described as being devoted to the clinical concerns of IVF. Related books written for the public by IVF advocates include the following from Australia: Peter Singer and Deane Wells, 1984; William Walters and Peter Singer (eds.), 1982; and Carl Wood and Ann Westmore, 1984.

Several sources on the history and practice of ultrasound in obstetrics appear in Chapter 4, note 1. Data and statistics from a variety of national and international studies of infertility appear in Chapter 4, note 3. These include World Health Organisation publications. Two medical articles on CVS are Elias, 1986 and Hogge *et al.*, 1986.

Two revealing books about the history of the first IVF birth are given in Chapter 5, note 3. One is by the IVF team Edwards and Steptoe, and the other is by Lesley and John Brown, the parents of Louise Brown.

Sources on social and cultural aspects of technology, mostly from a feminist perspective, appear in Chapter 5, note 5. Also interesting in Cynthia Cockburn's *The Machinery of Dominance: Women, Men and Technological Know How*, (1985) Pluto Press, London.

For a revealing article on the way scientists in Britain argued their way into the halls of political power in the Second World War, see Chapter 5, note 8.

A large bibliography of sources on genetics and eugenics appears in Daniel Kevles' *In the Name of Eugenics* (1985), and so I do not repeat them here. In chronicling the history and meaning of eugenics, I included the proceedings of the annual Eugenics Society Symposia in London (The Eugenics Society office is located at 69 Eccleston Square, London); see

Carter, 1983a; Benjamin *et al.*, 1974; Cox and Peel, 1972; Thoday and Parkes, 1968; Platt and Parkes, 1967. Also see some of the scientific views of eugenics in Clifford Grobstein, 1981; Luigi Cavalli-Sforza and Walter Bodmer, 1971, Julian Huxley, 1961; Frances Galton, 1883, 1889, 1892. Related to these is Erwin Schrödinger's *What is Life* (1944).

Many women have written about experiences of genetic screening; a few of these articles are listed in Chapter 6, note 4.

I used many scientific textbooks and articles (most from the above listed medical/science journals) on the principles of genetics and the methods of genetic engineering. They include the following which are not cited elsewhere in this book: Old and Primrose, 1985; Weatherall, 1984; Steel, 1984; Wolpert, 1984. I chose to include these, rather than others, because the Old and Primrose is popular among geneticists and the other three articles in *The Lancet* are relatively easy to understand for someone familiar with the basic scientific concepts of genetics (genes, DNA).

The International Biotechnology Directory 1985, mentioned in Chapter 6, note 7, is an invaluable guide to government and non-government organisations involved in biotechnology research and development.

For a list of the English language government reports on the NRTs, see the list of references, section (a); section (b) is a list of non-government reports I used, including those of medical/science bodies.

Two feminist sources on the birth control movement appear in Chapter 7, note 7. Books about the history of the contraceptive Pill by the pioneers themselves are Carl Djerassi, 1979; Gregory Pincus, 1965; John Rock, 1963; also see Paul Vaughan, 1970.

The ideology and practice of population control is discussed in many of the articles above. Also see Chapter 7, note 8 for two sources on the myth about 'Third World' dependency.

References

References are divided into sections: (a) government reports, (b) other reports, (c) books, articles and journals, (d) conferences, (e) oral references.

Abbreviations: (C) designates correspondence to a journal

BMJ = *British Medical Journal*
MRC = Medical Research Council
Nature = *Nature, London*
RCOG = Royal College of Obstetricians and Gynaecologists

(a) Government reports

Committee of Inquiry into Human Fertilisation and Embryology, *Report* (1984) HMSO, London. (Reprinted in Mary Warnock (1985) *A Question of Life*, Basil Blackwell, Oxford.

Department of Health and Social Security (1986) *Legislation on Human Infertility Services and Embryo Research: A Consultation Paper*, HMSO, London.

Ethics Advisory Board (1979) *Report and Conclusions: HEW Support of Research Involving Human* In Vitro *Fertilisation and Embryo Transfer*, Department of Health, Education and Welfare (US). (Reprinted in Clifford Grobstein (1981) *From Chance to Purpose*, Addison-Wesley, London.)

Genetisk Integritet. SOU 1984:88. English summary (1984) Liber Tryck, Stockholm, pp. 20–6. (The reference identifies Genetic Integrity as the Swedish Government's 88th official investigation in 1984.)

House of Representatives (US). Committee on Science and Technology, Subcommittee on Investigations and Oversights. *Hearing Report on Human Embryo Transfer held 9–10 August 1984*, US Government Printing Office, Washington DC (40–8000).

Ontario Law Reform Commission (1985) *Report on Human Artificial Reproduction and Related Matters*, Ministry of the Attorney General, Ontario. (Available from Publications Services Section, 5th Floor, 880 Bay Street, Toronto, Ontario M7A 1N8, Canada.)

220

Victoria, Committee to Consider the Social, Ethical and Legal Issues Arising from *In Vitro* Fertilisation. (a) 1982, *Interim Report*. (b) 1983, *Issues Paper on Donor Gametes in IVF*. (c) 1983, *Report on Donor Gametes in IVF*. (d) 1984, *Report on the Dispositions of Embryos Produced by* In Vitro *Fertilisation*.
Waller Report *see* Victoria, Committee to Consider.
Warnock Report *see* Committee of Inquiry.

(b) Other reports

American Fertility Society Ethics Committee (1986) 'Ethical Considerations of the New Reproductive Technologies', *Fertility and Sterility*, Supplement 1, Vol. 46, No. 3.
Council for Science and Society (1984) *Human Procreation*, London.
European Medical Research Councils' Subgroup on Human Reproduction (1984) 'Recommendations for Priority Areas in Human Reproduction Research', *The Lancet*, vol. 1:1228–30.
Jones, Alun and Walter Bodmer (1974) *Our Future Inheritance: Choice or Chance?* A Study by a British Association for the Advancement of Science Working Party, Committee on Science and Public Affairs, Oxford University Press, Oxford.
MRC (1984–5) *MRC Annual Report*, London.
MRC (1985) *Report of Inquiry into Human Fertilisation and Embryology: Medical Research Council Response*, London.
MRC/RCOG Voluntary Licensing Authority for Human *In Vitro* Fertilisation and Embryology (1985) *Guidelines for Both Clinical and Research Applications of Human* In Vitro *Fertilisation*.
MRC/RCOG Voluntary Licensing Authority for Human *In Vitro* Fertilisation and Embryology (1986) *The First Report of the Voluntary Licensing Authority for Human* In Vitro *Fertilisation and Embryology*.
MRC/RCOG Voluntary Licensing Authority for Human *In Vitro* Fertilisation and Embryology (1987) *The Second Report of the Voluntary Licensing Authority for Human* In Vitro *Fertilisation and Embryology*.
RCOG (1983) *Report of the RCOG Ethics Committee on* In Vitro *Fertilisation and Embryo Replacement or Transfer*, London.
RCOG *et al.* (1985) *Report on Fetal Viability and Clinical Practice*, London.
The Royal Society (1983) *Human Fertilisation and Embryology*. Submission to the Department of Health and Social Security Committee of Inquiry, London.
Science and Engineering Research Council (1986) *Science Board Research Themes*, SERC.

(c) Books, articles and journals

Agarwal, Anil (1979) 'More Babies Needed', *New Scientist*, 22 February, p. 591.

Akhter, Farida (1986a) 'Contraceptive Technology and the Coercive Reorganization of Society', unpublished paper from UBINIG, 5/3 Barabo Mahanpur Ring Road, Shaymoli, Dhaka-7.

Akhter, Farida (1986b) 'Depopulating Bangladesh: A Brief History of the External Intervention into the Reproductive Behaviour of a Society', UBINIG, Dhaka.

Akhter, Farida (1987) 'Wheat for Statistics: A Case Study of Relief Wheat for Attaining Sterilisation Target in Bangladesh', in Spallone and Steinberg (eds) *Made to Order*, Pergamon, Oxford.

American Medical News (1986) 'Parentage Decided for Unborn Child', 4 April, p. 17.

Anderson, Ian (1985) 'How IUDs Cause Infertility', *New Scientist*, 18 April, p. 6.

Anderson, W. French (1984) 'Prospects for Human Gene Therapy', *Science*, Vol. 226, pp. 401–9.

Andrews, Lori B. (1986) 'My Body, My Property', *Hastings Centre Report*, October, pp. 28–38.

Angell, R. *et al.* (1983) 'Chromosome Abnormalities in Human Embryos after IVF', *Nature*, Vol. 303, pp. 336–8.

'Appropriate Technology for Birth' (World Health Organisation Conference) (1985) *The Lancet*, vol. 2, pp. 436–87.

Arditti, Rita (1987) ' "Surrogate Mothering" Exploits Women', *Science for the People*, vol. 19, no. 3, pp. 22–3.

Arditti, Rita, Renate D. Klein and Shelley Minden (eds) (1984) *Test Tube Women: What Future for Motherhood*, Pandora, London.

Association of Radical Midwives (1986) The Vision: Proposals for the Future of Maternity Services, published by ARM, 62 Greetby Hill, Ormskirk, Lancs.

Austin, Colin R. (ed.) (1973) *The Mammalian Fetus In Vitro*, Chapman & Hall, London.

Barinaga, Marcia (1987) 'Field Test of Ice-minus Bacteria Goes Ahead Despite Vandals', *Nature*, vol. 326, p. 819.

Beardmore, John A. (1974) 'Some Genetic Consequences and Problems of the New Biology', in Benjamin *et al.* (eds) *Population and the New Biology*, Academic Press, London.

Beardsely, Tim (1985) 'Problems of Prenatal Testing', *Nature*, vol. 314, p. 211.

Benjamin, Bernard, Peter R. Cox and John Peel (eds) (1974) *Population and the New Biology*, Proceedings of the Tenth Annual Symposium of the Eugenics Society London, 1973, Academic Press, London.

Berger, John (1980) *About Looking*, Writers and Readers Cooperative, London.

Bertell, Rosalie (1985) *No Immediate Danger: Prognosis for a Radioactive Earth*, The Woman's Press, London.

Bleier, Ruth (1984) *Science and Gender*, Pergamon, New York.

Bodmer, Walter F. and Luigi Luca Cavalli-Sforza (1970) 'Intelligence and Race', *Scientific American*, vol. 223, no. 4, pp. 19–29.

Bodmer, Walter F. (1981) 'Gene Clusters, Genome Organization, and

Complex Phenotypes. When the Sequence is Known, What Will It Mean?' The William Allan Memorial Award Address, *American Journal of Human Genetics*, vol. 33, pp. 664–82.

Boler, Leo R. and Norbert Gleicher (1985) 'Maternal versus Fetal Rights', in Gleicher (ed.) *Principles of Medical Therapy in Pregnancy*, Plenum Medical Book Co., New York.

Boseley, Sarah (1987) 'Ex-prostitute Says Doctors Unfair on Test-Tube Baby', *The Guardian*, 21 October.

Bowes, Watson A. and Brad Selgestad (1981) 'Fetal Versus Maternal Rights: Medical and Legal Perspectives', *Obstetrics and Gynaecology*, vol. 58, no. 2, pp. 209–14.

Bradish, Paula (1987) 'From Genetic Counselling and Genetic Analysis to Genetic Ideal and Genetic Fate?' in Spallone and Steinberg (eds) *Made to Order*, Pergamon, Oxford.

Brahams, Diana (1983) '*In-vitro* Fertilisation and Related Research: Why Parliament Must Legislate', *The Lancet*, 14 September, pp. 726–9.

Breaking Chains (1986) 'Fetal Neglect Ruling', vol. 44.

Brinster, Ralph L. *et al.* (1982) 'Regulation of Metallothionein-thymidine Kinase Fusion Plasmid Injected into Mouse Eggs', *Nature*, vol. 296, pp. 39–42.

BMJ (1978) 'The Nulliparous Patient, the IUD, and Subsequent Infertility', vol. 2, p. 233.

BMJ (1983) 'Appendix VI: Interim Report on Human *In Vitro* Fertilisation and Embryo Replacement', vol. 286, pp. 1594–5.

BMJ (1985) 'BMA apologises to Mr Robert Edwards', vol. 291, p. 418.

Brown, Lesley and John Brown with Sue Freeman (1979) *Our Miracle Called Louise*, Paddington Press, New York.

Browne, Stephen (C) (1982) *BMJ*, vol. 285, pp. 1114–15.

Bullard, Linda (1987) 'Killing Us Softly: Toward a Feminist Analysis of Genetic Engineering', in Spallone and Steinberg (eds) *Made to Order*, Pergamon, Oxford.

Burfoot, Annette (1987) 'The Organisation and Normalisation of Reproductive Control', unpublished paper from the Annual Meeting of the British Sociological Association, 6–9 April, Leeds.

Campbell, Beatrix (1984) 'Why Didn't They Ask Women?' *The Guardian*, 7 November.

Carter, Cedric O. (1968) 'Conclusion', in Thoday and Parkes (eds) *Genetic and Environmental Influences and Behaviour*, Plenum Press, New York.

Carter, Cedric O. (1972) 'The New Eugenics?' The Galton Lecture 1971, in Cox and Peel (eds) *Population and Pollution*, Academic Press, London.

Carter, Cedric O. (ed.) (1983a) *Developments in Human Reproduction and their Eugenic, Ethical Implications.* Proceedings of the Nineteenth Annual Symposium of the Eugenics Society London 1982, Academic Press, London.

Carter, Cedric O. (1983b) Preface, in Carter (ed.) (1983a) *Developments in Human Reproduction*, Academic Press, London.

Carter, Cedric O. (1983c) 'Eugenic Implications of New Techniques', in

Carter (ed.) (1983a) *Developments in Human Reproduction*, Academic Press, London.

Cavalli-Sforza, Luigi L. and Walter F. Bodmer (1971) *The Genetics of Human Populations*, W. H. Freeman, San Francisco.

Chargaff, Erwin (1987) 'Engineering a Molecular Nightmare', *Nature*, vol. 327, pp. 199–200.

Chetley, Andrew (1986) *The Politics of Baby Food: Successful Challenges to an International Marketing Strategy*, Frances Pinter, London.

Cinque, Thomas J. (1987) 'Another Triangle: Mother, Doctor, and Fetus', *Hospital Physician*, December, pp. 67–8.

Clark, Ronald W. (1980) *The Greatest Power on Earth: The Story of Nuclear Fission*, Sidgwick & Jackson, London.

Clarke, Maxine (1985a) 'British Commons Vote for Ban', *Nature*, vol. 313, p. 618.

Clarke, Maxine (1985b) 'Voluntary Authority Set Up', *Nature*, vol. 314, p. 397.

Clarke, Maxine (1985c) 'Chances of Legislation Fade', *Nature*, vol. 318, p. 197.

Clarke, Maxine (1986) 'Another Bill Bites the Dust', *Nature*, vol. 319, p. 349.

Connor, Steve (1985) 'Scientists Licensed to Work on "pre-embryos",' *New Scientist*, 21 November, p. 21.

Coombs, J. (1985) *The International Biotechnology Directory*, Macmillan, London.

Corea, Gena (1985) *The Mother Machine*, Harper & Row, New York.

Corea, Gena et al. (1985) *Man-Made Women*, Hutchinson, London.

Corea, Gena and Susan Ince (1987) 'Report of a Survey of IVF Clinics in the US', in Spallone and Steinberg (eds) *Made to Order*, Pergamon, Oxford.

Cox, Peter and John Peel (1972) *Population and Pollution*. Proceedings of the Eighth Annual Symposium of the Eugenics Society London, 1971, Academic Press, London.

Cross, Michael (1986) 'Physicists Probe Ultrasound's Safety', *New Scientist*, 17 April, p. 27.

Crowe, Christine (1985) 'The Reproductive Fix', *Australian Left Review*, no. 91, pp. 4–9.

Crowe, Christine (1987a) 'Women Want It: *In Vitro* Fertilisation and Women's Motivations for Participation', in Spallone and Steinberg (eds) *Made to Order*, Pergamon, London.

Crowe, Christine (1987b) 'IVF, Scientific Knowledge and the Reproduction of Social Order', unpublished paper from the Annual Meeting of the British Sociological Association, 6–9 April, Leeds.

*Current Contents*1 (1984) 'Funding the New Origins of Life', vol. 52, p. 13. (Quoted from Claudia Wallis (1984) *Time*, 10 September, pp. 46–53.)

Daly, Mary (1979) *Gyn/Ecology: The Metaethics of Radical Feminism*, The Women's Press, London.

d'Arcy, Kim (1986) 'Super Pill Research', *Yorkshire Evening Press*, 17 June.

Davies, David (C) (1986) *Nature*, vol. 320, p. 208.

Davies, Saffron (1986) 'A Tall Story of Designer Genes', *The Guardian*, 29 November.

Davin, Anna (1978) 'Imperialism and Motherhood', *History Workshop*, Spring, pp. 9–69.

Dean, Malcolm (1986) 'Lords Uphold Ruling on Addict's Baby', *The Guardian*, 5 December.

Degener, Theresia (1986a) 'The Northern California Sperm Bank', unpublished paper presented at the First European Women's Conference on Reproductive and Genetic Engineering, Palma, 12 October.

Degener, Theresia (1986b) 'Prenatal Diagnosis – Sense and Nonsense', unpublished paper presented at the European Women's Conference on Reproductive and Genetic Engineering, Palma, 13 October.

Denning, John (1985) 'The Hazards of Women's Work', *New Scientist*, 17 January, pp. 12–15.

Diczfalusy, Egon (1986) World Health Organisation Special Programme of Research, Development and Research Training in Human Reproduction. 'The First Fifteen Years: A Review', *Contraception*, vol. 34, no. 1. Special issue.

Direcks, Anita (1987) 'Has the Lesson Been Learned? The DES story and IVF', in Spallone and Steinberg (eds) *Made to Order*, Pergamon, Oxford.

Dixon, Robyn (1985) 'Humans Could be a "Different Species"', conference told', *The Age*, 17 October.

Djerassi, Carl (1979) *The Politics of Contraception*, W. H. Freeman, San Francisco.

Drug and Therapeutics Bulletin (1985) 'Ultrasound in Pregnancy: Should It Be Routine?' vol. 23, no. 15, pp. 57–60.

Dunn, Elizabeth (1984) 'Meddling With the Conceptus', *The Sunday Times*, 25 November.

Dunstan, Gordon (1983) 'Social and Ethical Aspects', in Carter (ed.) (1983a), *Developments in Human Reproduction*, Academic Press, London.

Durant, John (1984) 'The Battle With Human Nature', *The Guardian*, 15 November.

Durant, John (1987) 'Vital Fugue' (book review), *Times Higher Education Supplement*, 13 March, p. 19.

Dworkin, Andrea (1983) *Right Wing Women*, The Women's Press, London.

Edwards, Robert G. (1957) 'The Experimental Induction of Gynogenesis in the Mouse. I: Irradiation of Sperm by X-rays'; and 'II: Ultraviolet Irradiation of the Sperm', *Proceedings of the Royal Society*, B, vol. 146, pp. 469–87, 488–504.

Edwards, Robert G. (1962) 'Meiosis in Ovarian Oocytes of Adult Mammals', *Nature*, vol. 196, pp. 446–50.

Edwards, Robert G. (1965) 'Maturation *in vitro* of Human Ovarian Oocytes', *The Lancet*, 6 November, pp. 926–9.

Edwards, Robert G. (1974) 'Fertilisation of Human Eggs *In Vitro*: Morals, Ethics and the Law', *Quarterly Review of Biology*, vol. 49, pp. 3–26.

Edwards, Robert G. (1980a) *Conception in the Human Female*, Academic Press, London.

Edwards, Robert G. (1980b) 'The Control Dish', in Edwards and Steptoe, *A Matter of Life*, Hutchinson, London.

Edwards, Robert G. (1980c) 'Farewell to Oldham', in Edwards and Steptoe, *A Matter of Life*, Hutchinson, London.

Edwards, Robert G. (1980d) 'The Shindy in Washington', in Edwards and Steptoe, *A Matter of Life*, Hutchinson, London.

Edwards, Robert G. (1983a) 'The Current Clinical and Ethical Situation of Human Conception *In Vitro*: The Galton Lecture 1982', in Carter (ed.) *Development in Human Reproduction*, Academic Press, London.

Edwards, Robert G. (1983b) 'Chromosome Abnormalities in Human Embryos', *Nature*, vol. 303, p. 283.

Edwards, Robert G., B. D. Bavistar and Patrick C. Steptoe (1969) 'Early Stages of Fertilisation *In Vitro* of Human Oocytes', *Nature*, vol. 221, pp. 632–5.

Edwards, Robert G., Roger P. Donahue, Theodore A. Baramki and Howard W. Jones (1966) 'Preliminary Attempts to Fertilise Human Oocytes Matured *In Vitro*', *American Journal of Obstetrics and Gynaecology* vol. 96, pp. 192–200.

Edwards, Robert G. and Margaret Puxon (1984) 'Parental Consent Over Embryos', *Nature*, vol. 310, p. 524.

Edwards, Robert G. and David J. Sharpe (1971) 'Social Values and Research in Human Embryology', *Nature*, vol. 231, pp. 87–91.

Edwards, Robert G., Patrick C. Steptoe and Jean M. Purdy (1970) 'Fertilisation and Cleavage *In Vitro* of Preovulatory Mature Oocytes', *Nature*, vol. 227, pp. 1307–9.

Edwards, Robert G. and Patrick C. Steptoe (1980) *A Matter of Life*, Hutchinson, London.

Edwards, Robert G. and Patrick C. Steptoe (1983) 'Current Status of *In Vitro* Fertilisation and Implantation of Human Embryos', *The Lancet*, 3 December, pp. 1265–9.

Ehrenreich, Barbara and Deirdre English (1979) *For Her Own Good: 150 Years of Experts' Advice to Women*, Pluto, London.

Elias, Sherman and George J. Annas (1983) 'Perspectives on Fetal Surgery', *American Journal of Obstetrics and Gynaecology*, vol. 145, no. 7. pp. 807–12.

Elias, Sherman and George J. Annas (1986) 'Social Policy Considerations in Noncoital Reproduction', *Journal of the American Medical Association*, vol. 255, no. 1, pp. 62–8.

Elias, Sherman *et al.* (1986) 'Chorionic Villus Sampling in Continuing Pregnancies, I: Low Fetal Loss Rates in Initial 109 Cases', *American Journal of Obstetrics and Gynaecology*, vol. 154, pp. 1349–52.

Elkington, John (1986) *The Poisoned Womb: Human Reproduction in a Polluted World*, Penguin, Harmondsworth.

Emery, Alan E. H. (1968) *Genetics in Medicine*. University of Edinburgh Inaugural Lecture, no. 35, University of Edinburgh.

Evans, H. John and Anne McLaren (1985) 'Unborn Children (Protection) Bill', *Nature*, vol. 314, pp. 127–8.

Finger, Anne (1984) 'Claiming All of Our Bodies: Reproductive Rights and Disabilities', in Arditti *et al.* (eds) *Test-Tube Women*, Pandora, London.

FINRRAGE (Feminist International Network of Resistance to Reproductive and Genetic Engineering) Holds proceedings of FINRRAGE conferences and international collection of newsclippings and articles. P.O. Box 587, London NW3.

Fleming, R. *et al.* (1985) 'Blockade of the LH Surge and Direct Control of Ovarian Function in Women with Functioning Pituitaries', in Rowland *et al.* (eds) *Gamete Quality and Fertility Regulation*, Excerpta Medica, Amsterdam.

Fletcher, John C. (1981) 'The Fetus as Patient: Ethical Issues', *Journal of the American Medical Association*, vol. 246, no. 7, pp. 772–3.

Foley, Gerald with Charlotte Nassim (1976) *The Energy Question*, Pelican, London.

'For and Against': The Essence of the Arguments as They Appeared in the Press (1982) in Walters and Singer (eds) *Test-Tube Babies*, Oxford University Press, Melbourne.

Forman, R., Simon B. Fishel, Robert G. Edwards and E. Walters (1985) 'The Influence of Transient Hyperprolactinemia on *in Vitro* Fertilisation in Humans', *Journal of Clinical Endocrinology and Metabolism*, vol. 60, pp. 517–22.

Franklin, Sarah (1987) 'The Social Construction of Infertility: Implications for Discussion of the New Reproductive Technologies', unpublished paper from The Annual Meeting of the British Sociological Association, Leeds, 6–9 April.

Frauen Gegen Gentechnik und Reproduktionstechnik. Dokumentation zum Kongreß vom 19–21.4.1985 in Bonn (1986) Verlag Kölner Volksblatt, Köln.

Free, Michael J. and Duncan, G. W. (1974) 'New Technology for Voluntary Sterilisation', in Benjamin *et al.* (eds) *Population and the New Biology*, Academic Press, London.

Galton, Francis (1883) *Inquiries Into Human Faculty*, Macmillan, London.

Galton, Francis (1889) *Natural Inheritance*, Macmillan, London.

Galton, Francis (1892) *Hereditary Genius*, Macmillan, London.

Garcia, Celso-Ramon *et al.* (eds) (1984) *Current Therapy of Infertility*, Decker, Philadelphia.

Garcia, Christina and Gregory H. Wierzynski (1985) 'Conquering Inherited Enemies', *Sun Herald*, Sydney, 20 October.

Gelman, David and Daniel Shapiro (1985) 'Infertility: Babies by Contract', *Newsweek*, 4 November, pp. 74–7.

GeneWATCH, Bulletin of the Committee for Responsible Genetics, 5 Doane St., Boston, MA 02109 (US).

Glatt, Jack (C) (1982) *BMJ*, vol. 285, p. 1355.

Gleicher, Norbert (ed.) (1985) *Principles of Medical Therapy in Pregnancy*, Plenum Medical Book Co., New York.

Gordon, Linda (1974) *Women's Body, Women's Right: A Social History of Birth Control in America*, Penguin, Harmondsworth.

Greenfeld, Dorothy and Florence Haseltine (1986) 'Candidate Selection and Psychosocial Considerations of In-Vitro Fertilisation Procedures', *Clinical Obstetrics and Gynaecology*, vol. 29, no. 1, pp. 119–26.

Grobstein, Clifford (1981) *From Chance to Purpose: An Appraisal of External Human Fertilisation*, Addison-Wesley, London.

Grobstein, Clifford (C) (1985) *Nature*, vol. 314, p. 666.

Grobstein, Clifford, Michael Flower, and John Mendeloff (1985) 'Frozen Embryos: Policy Issues', *New England Journal of Medicine*, vol. 312, no. 24, pp. 1584–8.

The Guardian (1985) 'Test-tube Baby Pioneer Wins Libel Apology from the BMA', 30 July.

The Guardian (1987a) 'Genetic Dab Hand', 7 January.

The Guardian (1987b) 'Genie in the Bottle', 13 June.

The Guardian (1987c) 'AIDS Technique Has Potential of Producing People to Order', 26 August.

The Guardian (1987d) 'Prenatal Test Could Eliminate Hare Lip', 27 August.

Guatemala Committee for Human Rights (1987) 'Health Care and Hope in Guatemala' (news sheet), GCHR, London.

Hammer, Robert E. *et al*. (1984) 'Partial Correction of Murine Hereditary Growth Disorder by Germ-line Incorporation of a New Gene', *Nature*, vol. 311, 65–7.

Hammer, Robert E. *et al*. (1985a) 'Expression of Human Growth Hormone-releasing Factor in Transgenic Mice Results in Increased Somatic Growth', *Nature*, vol. 315, pp. 413–16.

Hammer, Robert E. *et al*. (1985b) 'Production of Transgenic Rabbits, Sheep and Pigs by microinjection', *Nature*, vol. 315, pp. 680–2.

Hanmer, Jalna (1981) 'Sex Predetermination, Artificial Insemination and the Maintenance of Male-dominated Culture', in Helen Roberts (ed.) *Women, Health and Reproduction*, Routledge & Kegan Paul, London.

Hanmer, Jalna (1985) 'Transforming Consciousness: Women and the New Reproductive Technologies', in Corea *et al*. *Man-Made Women*, Hutchinson, London.

Hanmer, Jalna (1986) 'Locating Women in Reproductive and Genetic Engineering: Issues for Medical Sociology', *Medical Sociology News*, vol. 12, no. 1, pp. 6–21.

Harding, Sandra (1986) *The Science Question in Feminism*, Cornell University Press, Ithaca, New York.

Harris, Margaret (1985) 'Altering Genes in Unborn Babies', *Sydney Morning Herald*, 8 June.

Hartmann, Betsy (1987) 'A Womb of One's Own', *Science for the People*, vol. 19, no. 4, pp. 9–12.

Hastings Centre Report. Journal of the Institute of Society, Ethics and the Life Sciences, 360 Broadway, Hastings-on-Hudson, NY 10706 (US).

Hemsworth, B. N. (1974) 'The Creation of Life by New Means', in Benjamin *et al*. (eds) *Population and the New Biology*, Academic Press, London.

Hogge, W. Allen *et al.* (1986) 'Chorionic Villus Sampling: Experience of the First 1000 Cases', *American Journal of Obstetrics and Gynaecology*, vol. 154, pp. 1249–52.

Hopkins, Ellen (1985) 'High Tech Pregnancies', *The Newsday Magazine*, 11 August.

Hospitals (1985) 'Parents Choose Infant Gender at 28 Clinics', 16 September.

Hubbard, Ruth (1982) 'Legal and Policy Implications of Recent Advances in Prenatal Diagnosis and Fetal Therapy', *Women's Rights Law Reporter*, vol. 7, no. 2, pp. 201–18.

Hubbard, Ruth (1984) 'Personal Courage Is Not Enough: Some Hazards of Childbearing in the 1980s', in Arditti *et al.* (eds) *Test-Tube Women*, Pandora, London.

Hubbard, Ruth (1985) 'Prenatal Diagnosis and Eugenic Ideology', *Women's Studies International Forum*, vol. 8, no. 6, pp. 567–76.

Huggins, George R. (1984) 'Contraceptive Use and Future Reproductive Implications', in Garcia *et al.* (eds) *Current Therapy of Infertility*, Decker, Philadelphia.

Hunt, Mortan (1986) 'The Total Gene Screen', *The New York Times Magazine*, 19 January, p. 33ff.

Huntingford, Peter (C) (1979) *BMJ*, vol. 2, p. 496.

Huws, Ursula (1987) *VDU Hazards Handbook: A Workers Guide to the Effects of New Technology*, London Hazards Centre Trust, London.

Huxley, Andrew (1985) Research and the Embryo. *New Scientist*, 11 April, p. 2.

Huxley, Julian (ed.) (1961a) *The Humanist Frame*, George Allen & Unwin, London.

Huxley, Julian (1961b) 'The Humanist Frame', in Huxley (ed.) *The Humanist Frame*, George Allen & Unwin, London.

Hynes, H. Patricia (1987) 'A Paradigm for the Regulation of the Biomedical Industry: Environmental Protection in the United States', in Spallone and Steinberg (eds) *Made to Order*, Pergamon, Oxford.

International Report (1987) in Spallone and Steinberg (eds) *Made to Order*, Pergamon, Oxford.

Ironside, Virginia (1985) 'How to Breed Healthy Babies', *The Guardian*, 18 November.

Jacobs, H. S. *et al.* (1985) 'Endocrine Control of Follicular Growth in Humans', Reinier de Graaf Lecture, in Rowland *et al.* (eds) *Gamete Quality and Fertility Regulation*, Excerpta Medica, Amsterdam.

Jansen, Sarah (1986) 'Eco-feminist Evaluation of the Techniques', in the documentation from the Women's Hearing on Genetic Engineering and Reproductive Technologies, Brussels, 6–7 March.

Japanese Women Struggling for Liberation (1984) Published by Asian Women's Association, Japanese Women's Caucus Against War, Japanese Women's Council, Group for Creating Equal Employment Opportunity Law, 82 Committee Against Revision of Eugenic Protection Law, Tokyo.

Johnston, Ian *et al.* (1981) '*In Vitro* Fertilisation: The Challenge of the Eighties', *Fertility and Sterility*, vol. 36, no. 6, pp. 699–705.

Johnston, Kathy (1987) 'Sex of New Embryos Known', *Nature*, vol. 327, p. 547.

Jones, Howard (1985) 'First World'. Special issue on new birth technologies, *Omni*, December, p. 6.

Journal of Medical Ethics. Quarterly started in 1975 by the Society for the Study of Medical Ethics, now Institute of Medical Ethics, Tavistock House North, Tavistock Square, London.

Joyce, Christopher (1987) 'Patents Law Protects Altered Organisms', *New Scientist*, 30 April, p. 27.

Kamal, Sultana (1987) 'Seizure of Reproductive Rights? A discussion on population control in the third world and the emergence of the new reproductive technologies in the West', in Spallone and Steinberg (eds) *Made to Order*, Pergamon, Oxford.

Kass, Leon R. (1971) 'Babies by Means of *In Vitro* Fertilisation: Unethical Experiments on the Unborn?' *New England Journal of Medicine*, vol. 285, pp. 1174–9.

Katsh, Seymour (1969) 'Immunological Aspects of Reproduction', in M. C. Shelesnyak and George J. Marcus (eds) *Ovum Implantation*. Proceedings held at the Weizmann Institute of Science, Tehovath, Israel. August 1967, Gordon & Breach, New York.

Katz, Jay (1980) 'Disclosure and Consent', in Milunsky and Annas (eds) *Genetics and the Law II*, Plenum, New York.

Kaufmann, Caroline L. and Paul R. Williams (1985) 'Fetal Surgery: The Social Implications of Medical and Surgical Treatment of the Unborn Child', *Women and Health*, vol. 10, no. 1, pp. 25–37.

Kee, Cynthia (1987) 'Any Immediate Danger?' *The Observer*, 17 May.

Kennedy, Ian and Robert G. Edwards (1975) 'A Critique of the Law Commission Report on Injuries to Unborn Children and the Proposed Congenital Disabilities (Civil Liability) Bill', *Journal of Medical Ethics*, Part I, pp. 116–21.

Kevles, Daniel J. (1985) *In the Name of Eugenics*, Knopf, New York.

Kishwar, Madhu (1985) 'The Continuing Deficit of Women in India and the Impact of Amniocentesis', in Corea *et al.*, *Man-Made Women*, Hutchinson, London.

Kitzinger, Sheila (1985) 'Battle of Birth Rights', *The Sunday Times*, 19 May.

Klein, Renate (1985) 'What's New About the New Technologies?' in Corea *et al.*, *Man-Made Women*, Hutchinson, London.

Klein, Renate (1986) 'IVF: For Whose Benefit – At whose expense?' unpublished paper presented at the European Conference of Critical Legal Studies: Feminist Perspectives on Law, 3–5 April, University of London.

Klein, Renate (ed.) (1989) forthcoming, *The Exploitation of Infertility: Women and Reproductive Technologies*, The Women's Press, London.

Koch, Lena and Janice Morgall (1987) 'Toward a Feminist Assessment of Reproductive Technology', *Acta Sociologica*, vol. 30, no. 2, pp. 173–91.

Koch, Sally (1985) 'Disagreement Over Treating Gravida Against Her Wishes', *Ob Gyn News*, vol. 20, no. 9, pp. 1, 20.

Kolder, Veronika E. B., Janet Gallagher and Michael T. Parsons (1987) 'Court-Ordered Obstetrical Interventions', *New England Journal of Medicine*, vol. 316, no. 19, pp. 1192–6.

Kolko, Joyce (1974) *America and the Crisis of World Capitalism*, Beacon, Boston.

Kuhse, Helge (1986) 'Ethical Issues in Reproductive Alternatives for Genetic Indications', abstract, 7th International Congress of Human Genetics, 22–26 September, Berlin (West).

Kuhse, Helge and Peter Singer (1985) *Should the Baby Live: The Problem of Handicapped Infants*, Oxford University Press, Oxford.

Laborie, Françoise (1986) 'Some Recent News from France', paper presented at the First European Women's Conference on Reproductive and Genetic Engineering, Palma.

Laborie, Françoise (1987) 'Looking for Mothers, You Only Find Fetuses', in Spallone and Steinberg (eds) *Made to Order*, Pergamon, Oxford.

Laborie, Françoise (1988) 'New Reproductive Technologies: New From France',*Reproductive and Genetic Engineering International Feminist Viewpoints*, vol. 1, no. 1.

Leeds Women's Reproductive Rights Campaign (1984) 'Response to the Report of the Committee of Inquiry into Human Fertilisation and Embryology', unpublished.

Lindenberg, S. *et al.* (1985) 'Ectopic Pregnancy and Spontaneous Abortions Following *in vitro* Fertilisation and Embryo Transfer', *Acta Obstet. Gynecol. Scand*, vol. 64, pp. 31–4.

Lopata, Alexander (1980) 'Successes and Failures in Human *in Vitro* Fertilisation', *Nature*, vol. 288, p. 642.

McCance, Robert A. (1973) 'The Road Ahead', in Austin (ed.) *The Mammalian Fetus In Vitro*, Chapman & Hall, London.

McCance, Robert A. (1977) 'Perinatal Physiology', in Alan Hodgkin *et al.*, *The Pursuit of Nature: Informal Essays on the History of Physiology*, Cambridge University Press, Cambridge.

McKie, Robin (1987) 'Birth Defect Discovery Hailed by Doctors', *The Observer*, 15 March.

McKusick, Victor A. (1964) *Human Genetics*, Prentice-Hall, Englewood Cliffs.

McLaren, Angus (1984) *Reproductive Rituals*, Methuen, London.

McLaren, Anne (1976) *Mammalian Chimeras*, Cambridge University Press, London.

McLaren, Anne (1986a) 'Why Study Early Human Development?', *New Scientist*, 24 April, pp. 49–52.

McLaren, Anne (C) (1986b) *Nature*, vol. 320, p. 570.

Macnaughton, Malcolm C. (1973) 'Extracorporeal Maintenance of Small Human Fetuses', in Austin (ed.) *The Mammalian Fetus In Vitro*, Chapman & Hall, London.

'Made in a Lab', panel addressing ethical and legal problems of IVF from the television series *Society, Science and Sex*, presented on Granada Television (UK), 12 May 1986 (transcript).

Marrs, Richard (C) (1984) *American Journal of Obstetrics and Gynaecology*, vol. 149, no. 2, p. 237.

Maternity Alliance (Britain) (1985) 'Benefit Proposals Put Babies Health At Risk', Maternity Alliance Press Release, December.

Medawar, Peter B. and Jean S. Medawar (1977) *The Life Science: Current Ideas of Biology*, Wildwood House, London.

Menkin, Miriam F. and John Rock (1948) '*In Vitro* Fertilisation and Cleavage of Human Ovarian Eggs', *American Journal of Obstetrics and Gynaecology*, vol. 55, pp. 440–52.

Merchant, Carolyn (1982) *The Death of Nature: Women, Ecology and the Scientific Revolution*, Wildwood House, London.

Meulenbelt, Anja, Joyce Outshoorn, Selma Sevenhuijsen and Petra de Vries (eds) (tr. Della Couling) (1984) *A Creative Tension*, Pluto, London.

Mezzacappa, Dale (1986) 'The New Motherhood: Science Creates Social Issues', *The Philadelphia Inquirer*, 22 June.

Midwives Chronicle & Nursing Notes (1986) Parliamentary Report, September, p. 207.

Mies, Maria (1981) *The Social Origins of the Sexual Division of Labour*. Occasional Paper No. 85, Institute of Social Studies, The Hague, The Netherlands.

Mies, Maria (1986) *Patriarchy and Accumulation on a World Scale*, Zed, London.

Mies, Maria (1987) 'Why Do We Need All This? A Call Against Genetic Engineering and Reproductive Technology', in Spallone and Steinberg (eds) *Made to Order*, Pergamon, Oxford.

Milunsky, Aubrey and George J. Annas (eds) (1980) *Genetics and the Law II*, Plenum, New York.

Morgan, Charles (1987) 'New Australian Law on Embryos Still Confuses Researchers', *Nature*, vol. 325, p. 185.

Moss, Timothy and Janet Hawkswell (1986) 'Evidence of Infection with Chlamydia Trachomatis in Patients with Pelvic Inflammatory Disease: Value of Partner Investigation', *Fertility and Sterility*, vol. 45, no. 3, pp. 429–30.

Muller, Hermann J. (1961) 'The Human Future', in Huxley (ed.) (1961a) *The Humanist Frame*, George Allen & Unwin, London.

Murray, Thomas H. (1985) 'Ethical Issues in Fetal Surgery', *American College of Surgeons Bulletin*, vol. 70, no. 6, pp. 6–10.

National Perinatal Statistics Unit (Sydney) (1987) 'In Vitro Fertilisation Pregnancies, Australia and New Zealand 1979–1985', Fertility Society of Australia.

Nature (1982) 'The Future of the Test Tube Baby', vol. 299, pp. 475–6.

Nature (1983) 'Embryology Needs Rules, Not New Laws', vol. 302, pp. 735–6.

Nature (1984) 'Artificial Fertilisation Made Natural', vol. 310, p. 269.

Nature (1985a) 'Surrogacy Falsely in the Dock', vol. 313, p. 83.

Nature (1985b) 'Warnock Proposals in Trouble', vol. 313, p. 417.

Nature (1985c) 'UK Agonizes on Embryo Research', vol. 313, p. 424.

Nature (1985d) 'Embryos untouched?' vol. 313, p. 612.

Nature (1986) 'Tough Talk on Surrogate Birth', vol. 320, p. 95.

Nature (1987) 'IVF Remains in Legal Limbo', vol. 327, p. 87.

Neilson, J. P. (1986) 'Indications for Ultrasonography in Obstetrics', *Birth*, vol. 13, no. 1, pp. 16–20.

New, Denis A. T. (1973) 'Studies on Mammalian Fetuses *in vitro* During the Period of Organogenesis', in Austin (ed.) *The Mammalian Fetus In Vitro*, Chapman & Hall, London.

New, Denis A. T. (1983) '*In Vitro* Culture of Embryo and Fetus', in Carter (ed.) (1983a) *Developments in Human Reproduction*, Academic Press, London.

New Scientist (1982a) 'Test-tube Babies Under the Microscope', 4 February, p. 290.

New Scientist (1982b) 'Italy's First Test-tube Baby', 1 July, p. 7.

New Scientist (1986a) 'Frozen Eggs Find Ethical Favour in Australia', 24 April, p. 22.

New Scientist (1986b) 'Chemical Clue to Huntingdon's Disease', 22 May, p.28.

Newmark, Peter (1986) 'Danger of Delay for Genetic Tests', *Nature*, vol. 321, p. 557.

Newmark, Peter (1987) 'DNA Fingerprinting at a Price at ICI's UK Laboratory', *Nature*, vol. 327, p. 548.

Newsome, John (1986) 'Test Case That Could End the Ethical Dispute', *Yorkshire Evening Press*, 26 August.

Nilsson, Annika and Cindy de Wit (1986) 'Genetic Integrity – Critique of a Swedish Report on the Application of Genetic Technology on Humans', from documentation of the Women's Hearing on Genetic Engineering and Reproductive Technologies, 6–7 March, Brussels.

Nixon, D. A. (1973) 'Experimental Techniques in Fetal and Placental Physiology', in Austin (ed.) *The Mammalian Fetus In Vitro*, Chapman & Hall, London.

Oakley, Ann (1986) 'The History of Ultrasonography in Obstetrics', *Birth*, vol. 13, no. 1, pp. 8–13, paper presented at the Royal Society of Medicine Forum on Maternity and the Newborn: Ultrasonography in Obstetrics, 17 April 1985.

Ob Gyn News (1985a) '"Extra" Embryo Issue in *In Vitro* Fertilisation', vol. 20, no. 9, pp. 3, 19.

Ob Gyn News (1985b) 'Chorionic Villus Sampling May Live up to Its Promise', vol. 20, no. 9, p. 8.

O'Brien, Mary, (1981) *The Politics of Reproduction*, Routledge & Kegan Paul, London.

Old, R. W. and S. B. Primrose (1985) *Principles of Gene Manipulation: An Introduction to Genetic Engineering*, Blackwell Scientific Publications, Oxford.

Palca, Joseph (1986) 'Department of Energy on the Map', *Nature*, vol. 321, p. 371.

Palfreman, Jon (1986) 'What a Piece of Work Is Man', *The Listener*, 16 January, pp. 13–14.

Pappworth, Maurice Henry (1967) *Human Guinea Pigs: Experimentation on Man,* Routledge & Kegan Paul, London.

Paul, Diane B. (1986) 'The History of the Eugenics Movement and Its Multiple Effects on Public Policy (book review), *Scientific American,* January, pp. 18–21

Peel, John (C) (1979) *BMJ,* vol. 2, p. 495.

Peters, James A. (ed) (1959) *Classic Papers in Genetics,* Prentice-Hall, New Jersey.

Pfeffer, Naomi and Anne Woollett (1983) *The Experience of Infertility,* Virago, London.

Pfeiffer, Regina Asaph and Katherine Whitlock (1984) *Fertility Awareness,* Prentice-Hall, Englewood Cliffs.

Pincus, Gregory (1965) *The Control of Fertility,* Academic Press, New York.

Pincus, Gregory and E. V. Enzmann (1935) 'The Comparative Behaviour of Mammilian Eggs *in vitro* and *in vivo,* I: The Activation of Ovarian Eggs', *Journal of Experimental Medicine,* vol. 62, pp. 665–75.

Pittaway, Donald E. (C) (1984) *American Journal of Obstetrics and Gynaecology,* vol. 149, no. 2, p. 236.

Platt, Lord and Alan S. Parkes (eds) (1967) *Social and Genetic Influences on Life and Death.* A Symposium held by the Eugenics Society in September 1966, Oliver & Boyd, Edinburgh.

Prentice, Thomson (1984) 'Pioneers Defend Embryo Research', *The Times,* 19 December.

Radford, Tim and Andrew Veitch (1986) 'Gene Research Brings Help to Parents', *The Guardian,* 6 September.

Rakusen, Jill (1982) 'In Pursuit of the Perfect Baby', unpublished article. (Available from WRRIC, 52–4 Featherstone St, London. This piece was originally written for *Out of Our Hands: What Technology Does to Pregnancy* by Jill Rakusen and Nicky Davidson (1982) Pan. The publishers suppressed it.)

Rapp, Rayna (1984) 'XYLO: A True Story', in Arditti *et al.* (eds) *Test-Tube Women,* Pandorà, London.

Raymond, Janice G. (1987) 'Fetalists and Feminists: They Are Not the Same', in Spallone and Steinberg (eds) *Made to Order,* Pergamon, Oxford.

Rich, Adrienne (1976) *Of Women Born,* Bantam, Toronto.

Rich, Adrienne (1980) *On Lies, Secrets and Silence,* Virago, London.

Ridgeway, G. L. *et al.* (1983) 'Therapeutic Abortion and Chlamydial Infection', *BMJ,* vol. 286, pp. 1478–9.

Ridler, M. A. C. and M. S. Grewal (1984) 'Possible Sources of Error in Prenatal Diagnosis Via Chorionic Villus Biopsy', *BMJ,* 12 May, p. 1081.

Rifkin, Jeremy (1985) *Declaration of a Heretic,* Routledge & Kegan Paul, Boston.

Robertson, Miranda (1986) 'Desperate Appliances', *Nature,* vol. 320, pp. 213–14.

Robinson, Jean (1987) See list of oral references.

Rock, John (1963) *The Time Has Come: A Catholic Doctor's Proposals to End the Battle over Birth Control*, Knopf, New York.

Rothman, Barabara Katz (1984) 'The Meanings of Choice in Reproductive Technology', in Arditti *et al. (eds) Test-Tube Women*, Pandora, London.

Rothman, Babara Katz (1986) *The Tentative Pregnancy: Prenatal Diagnosis and the Future of Motherhood*, Viking, New York.

Rowland, George F. and Timothy R. Moss (1985) '*In Vitro* Fertilisation, Previous Ectopic Pregnancy, and Chlamydia Trachomatis Infection', *The Lancet,* 12 October, p. 830.

Rowland, George F. *et al.* (1985) 'Failure of *In Vitro* Fertilisation and Embryo Replacement Following Infection with Chlamydia Trachomatis', *Journal of In Vitro Fertilisation and Embryo Transfer*, vol. 2, no. 3, pp. 151–5.

Rowland, R. *et al.* (eds) (1985) *Gamete Quality and Fertility Regulation.* Proceedings of the Vth Reiner de Graaf Symposium, Nijmegen, The Netherlands, 23–25 August 1984, Excerpta Medica, Amsterdam.

Rowland, Robyn (1985) 'A Child at any Price? An Overview of the Issues and the Use of the New Reproductive Technologies and the Threat to Women', *Women's Studies International Forum*, vol. 8, no. 6, pp. 539–46.

Russell, Bertrand (1929) *Marriage and Morals,* reissued 1985, Unwin Paperbacks, London.

Sandow, J (1983) 'Clinical Applications of LHRH and Its Analogues', *Clinical Endocrinology*, vol. 18, pp. 571–92.

Sarkar, Salil, (1987) 'Genetic Engineering Banned', *Times Higher Education Supplement*, 9 January.

Saxton, Marsha (1984) 'Born and Unborn: The Implications of Reproductive Technologies for People with Disabilities', in Arditti *et al.* (eds) *Test-Tube Women*, Pandora, London.

Scientific American (1985) Issue devoted to 'The Molecules of Life', October.

Scientific American (1987) 'Policing Pregnancy', August, pp. 19–20.

Schrödinger, Erwin (1944) *What is Life?* Cambridge University Press, Cambridge.

Seaman, Barbara and Gideon Seaman (1978) *Women and the Crisis in Sex Hormones: An Investigation of the Dangerous Use of Hormones from Birth Control to Menopause and the Safe Alternatives*, Harvester. Hassocks, Sussex.

Sevenhuijsen, Selma and Petra de Vries (1984) 'The Women's Movement and Motherhood', in Meulenblatt *et al.* (eds) *A Creative Tension*, Pluto, London.

Sevenhuijsen, Selma and Jolande Withuis (1984) 'The Policing of Families', in Meulenblatt *et al.* (eds) *A Creative Tension,* Pluto, London.

7th International Congress of Human Genetics. Abstracts Part 1. (1986) 22–26 September, Berlin (West).

Sher, Geoffrey *et al.* (1984) 'The Development of a Successful Non-university-based Ambulatory *In Vitro* Fertilisation/Embryo Transfer Program: Phase 1', *Fertility and Sterility*, vol. 41, no. 4, pp. 511–18.

Shettles, Landrum B. (1955) 'A Morula Stage of Human Ovum Developed *In Vitro*', *Fertility and Sterility*, vol. 6, pp. 287–9.

Short, Roger V. (1981) 'Test Tube to Womb: Ethics and Politics' (book review) *Nature*, vol. 294, pp. 38–9.

Singer, Peter and Deane Wells (1984) *The Reproductive Revolution: New Ways of Making Babies*, Oxford University Press, Oxford.

Smith, Pricilla Kincaid (1982) 'The Ethics of *In Vitro* Fertilisation', *BMJ*, vol. 284, p. 1287.

Soules, Michael (1985) 'The *In Vitro* Fertilisation Pregnancy Rate: Let's Be Honest with One Another', *Fertility and Sterility*, vol. 43, no. 4, pp. 511–13.

Spallone, Patricia (1986) 'The Warnock Report: The Politics of Reproductive Technology', *Women's Studies International Forum*, vol. 9, no. 5, pp. 543–50.

Spallone, Patricia (1987) 'Reproductive Technology and the State: The Warnock Report and Its Clones', in Spallone and Steinberg (eds) *Made to Order*, Pergamon, Oxford.

Spallone, Patricia and Deborah Lynn Steinberg (eds) (1987) *Made to Order: The Myth of Reproductive and Genetic Progress*, Pergamon, Oxford.

Steel, C. M. (1984) 'DNA in Medicine. The Tools', *The Lancet*, 20 October, pp. 853–6.

Steinbacher, Roberta and Helen B. Holmes (1985) 'Sex Choice: Survival and Sisterhood', in Corea *et al.*, *Man-Made Women*, Hutchinson, London.

Steinberg, Deborah Lynn (1987) 'Selective Breeding and Social Engineering: Disciminatory Policies of Access to Artificial Insemination by Donor in Great Britain', in Spallone and Steinberg (eds), *Made to Order*, Pergamon, Oxford.

Steptoe, Patrick (1980a) 'If Only', in Edwards and Steptoe, *A Matter of Life*, Hutchinson, London.

Steptoe, Patrick (1980b) 'Birth of a Baby', in Edwards and Steptoe, *A Matter of Life*, Hutchinson, London.

Steptoe, Patrick C. and Robert G. Edwards (1970) 'Laparoscopic Recovery of Preovulatory Human Oocytes After Priming of Ovaries with Gonadotrophins', *The Lancet*, 4 April, pp. 683–9.

Steptoe, Patrick and Robert Edwards (C) (1983) *BMJ*, vol. 286, p. 1351.

Stewart, C. M. (1974) 'Population Policies in the Developing Countries', in Benjamin *et al.* (eds) *Population and the New Biology*, Academic Press, London.

Sullivan, Walter (1987a) 'Fetal Tissue Implants in Brain Seen', *The New York Times*, 1 July.

Sullivan, Walter (1987b) 'At N.Y.U., Pioneering Brain Surgery, *The New York Times*, 9 July.

Sunday Star Review (South Africa) (1985) 'Dora Plays Key Role in Biotechnology', 8 December.

Tate, Alan (1985) 'Fetal Tissue Transplants May Be Cure for Diabetes', *Sydney Morning Herald*, 6 July.

Taylor, Gordon Rattray (1968) *The Biological Time-Bomb,* Thames & Hudson, London.
Teichman, Jenny (1982) *Illegitimacy: A Philosophical Examination,* Basil Blackwell, Oxford.
Templeton, A. A. *et al.* 'What Potential Ovum Donors Think', *The Lancet,* 12 May, pp. 1081–2.
Thoday, John M. and Alan S. Parkes (1968) *Genetic and Environmental Influences on Behaviour.* A Symposium Held by the Eugenics Society in September 1967, Plenum Press, New York.
Thompson, Larry (1987) 'Brain Implants: The Controversial New Approach to Treating Parkinson's Disease', *Washington Post,* 14 July, pp. 12–17.
Time (1984) 'The New Origins of Life', 10 September, pp. 34–43.
Timmins, Nicholas (1985) 'BMA Fears Abortion Controversy', *The Times,* 22 July.
Tomasi, Ana M. and Bruce A. Work (1985) 'Diagnostic and Therapeutic Management of Fetal Disease', in Gleicher (ed.) *Principles of Medical Therapy in Pregnancy,* Plenum, New York.
Travis, Alan (1986) 'Blood Test for Immigrants', *The Guardian,* 29 October.
Trounson, Alan and Angelo Conti (1982) 'Research in Human *In Vitro* Fertilisation and Embryo Transfer, *BMJ,* vol. 285, pp. 244–8.
Trounson, Alan *et al.* (1983a) 'Pregnancy Established in an Infertile Patient After Transfer of a Donated Embryo Fertilised *In Vitro*', *BMJ,* vol. 286, pp. 835–8.
Trounson, Alan, Carl Wood and John Leeton (C) (1983b) *BMJ,* vol. 286, pp. 1351–2.
Turney, Jon (1985) 'Embryo Guidelines Set Out', *Times Higher Education Supplement,* 14 June.
UBINIG (undated) Policy Research for Development Alternative Information pamphlet. UBINIG 5/3 Barabo Mahanpur Ring Road, Shaymoli, Dhaka-7, Bangladesh.
Vaughan, Paul (1970) *The Pill on Trial,* Coward–McCann, New York.
Veitch, Andrew (1984a) 'Goddess of the Embryos', *The Guardian,* 22 May.
Veitch, Andrew (1984b) 'Scientists "Should Be Granted Use of Six-week embryos for research"', *The Guardian,* 24 May.
Veitch, Andrew (1985a) 'Embryo Tests Await Go-ahead', *The Guardian,* 19 November.
Veitch, Andrew (1985b) 'Cancer Team Wants Human Embryo Cells', *The Guardian,* 20 November.
Veitch, Andrew (1987a) 'Hospital Told to Stop Giving Eggs from Sisters to Infertile Women', *The Guardian,* 7 May.
Veitch, Andrew (1987b) 'Couples Will Be Able to Check "healthy" Embryos', *The Guardian,* 11 June.
Veitch, Andrew (1987c) 'Don't Strain NHS, Test Tube Baby Team Told', *The Guardian,* 13 June.
Veitch, Andrew (1987d) 'Doctors Fear World Trade in Stockpiled Embryos', *The Guardian,* 5 October.

238   *References*

Verp, Marion S. (1985) 'Genetic Counselling', in Gleicher (ed.) *Principles of Medical Therapy in Pregnancy*, Plenum, New York.
Vines, Gail (1987) 'Better Ways of Breeding', *New Scientist*, 13 August, pp. 51–4.
Von Ow, Barbara (1985) 'Eichmann Slur on Geneticists', *Times Higher Education Supplement*, 7 June.
Waddington, Conrad H. (1956) *Principles of Embryology*, George Allen & Unwin, London.
Waddington, Conrad H. (1961) 'The Human Animal', in Huxley (ed.) (1961a) *The Humanist Frame*, George Allen & Unwin, London.
Wagatsuma, Takashi (1981) 'New Developments in IDU's', in Chang Chai Fen and David Griffin (eds) *Recent Advances in Fertility Regulation*. Proceedings of a Symposium organised by the Ministry of Public Health of the People's Republic of China and the WHO's Special Programme of Research, Development and Research Training in Human Reproduction, Geneva.
Wallach, Edwards E. and Roger D. Kempers (eds) (1979) *Modern Trends in Infertility and Conception Control*, vol. 1, Williams & Wilkins, Baltimore.
Walmgate, Robert (1986) 'French Scientist Makes a Stand', *Nature*, vol. 323, p. 385.
Walsh, James B. and Jon Marks (C) (1986) *Nature*, vol. 322, p. 590.
Walsh, Vivien (1980) 'Contraception: The Growth of a Technology', in Brighton Women and Science Group, *Alice Through the Microscope*, Virago, London.
Walters, Leroy (1986) 'The Ethics of Human Gene Therapy', *Nature*, vol. 320, pp. 225–7.
Walters, William and Peter Singer (eds) (1982) *Test-Tube Babies*, Oxford University Press, Melbourne.
Weatherall, David J. (1984) 'DNA in Medicine: Implications for Medical Practice and Human Biology', *The Lancet*, 22 December, pp. 1440–4.
Weatherall, David J. (1985) *The New Genetics and Clinical Practice*, Oxford University Press, Oxford.
Weekend Australian (1986) 'Geneticists Give Farmers the Instant Pig', 1–2 February.
Wilkins, Maurice (1986) 'Science, Peace and Life', *New Scientist*, 13 March, pp. 48–9.
Wilkinson, James (1982) 'Human Embryo Furore', *New Scientist*, 14 October, pp. 115–16.
Williams, Peter and Gordon Stevens (1982) 'What Now for Test-tube Babies', *New Scientist*, 4 February, pp. 312–16.
Winslade, William J. (1981) 'Surrogate Mothers: Private Right or Public Wrong?' *Journal of Medical Ethics*, vol. 7, pp. 153–4.
Winston, Robert (1985) 'Why We Need to Experiment', *The Observer*, 10 February.
Wolpert, Lewis (1984) 'DNA in Medicine', *The Lancet*, 13 October, pp. 853–6.
Women's Reproductive Rights Information Centre (undated) Depo Provera (information sheet). WRRIC, 52 Featherstone Street, London.

Women's World, (Isis/WICCE) (1986) 'Appropriate Technology Following Birth', vol. 12, p. 36.
Wood, Carl and Ann Westmore (1984) *Test Tube Conception,* George Allen & Unwin, London.
Wood, Carl *et al.* (1984) 'Clinical Implications of Developments in *In Vitro* Fertilisation', *BMJ,* vol. 289, pp. 978–81.
Wood, Clive (1974) 'The Future of Oral Contraceptives', in Benjamin *et al. Population and the New Biology,* Academic Press, London.
World Health Organisation Fourteenth Annual Report. 1985. Special Programme of Research, Development and Research Training in Human Reproduction, Geneva.
Wright, Pierce (1978) 'Birth Is the Fruit of Years of Study', *The Times,* 27 July.
Yanchinski, Stephanie (1982) 'Research on Embryos: Ethics Under Fire', *New Scientist,* 30 September, p. 891.
Yovich, John *et al.* (1982) '*In Vitro* Fertilisation Pregnancy with Early Progestagen Support', *The Lancet,* 14 August, p. 378.
Yovich, John *et al.* (1983) 'Medroxyprogesterone in *In-vitro* Fertilisation', *The Lancet,* 26 March, p. 711.

(d) Conferences

Women's Emergency Conference on the New Reproductive Technologies, 3–8 July 1985, Vällinge.
Women's Hearing on Genetic Engineering and Reproductive Technologies at the European Parliament, 6–7 March 1986, Brussels.
European Conference of Critical Legal Studies: Feminist Perspectives on Law, 3–5 April 1986, London.
European Women's Conference on Reproductive Technology and Genetic Engineering, 11–15 October 1986, Palma.
Women, Reproduction and Technology, 14–15 February 1987, History Workshop Centre, Oxford.

(e) Oral references

BBC Radio 4 (1986) 'A Very Superior Baby', British Broadcasting Corporation, 9 January.
Discussion with Anne McLaren, FRS, Director of the Medical Research Council Mammalian Development Unit and member of the British Committee of Inquiry into Human Fertilisation and Embryology, on 15 February 1987, in Oxford.
Discussion with Professor Jerome Strauss, Department of Obstetrics and Gynaecology and Director, Division of Reproductive Biology, University of Pennsylvania (US) on 31 December 1985, in Philadelphia.
Leese, Henry (1986) '*In Vitro* Fertilisation and Embryo Transfer', lecture at the 1986 Annual Meeting of the Association for Science Education, University of York, 4 January.

Robinson, Jean (1987) 'Sexual Bias in Cervical Cancer Screening', presentation at Women, Reproduction and Technology conference, 15 February.

Steptoe, Patrick (1987) '*In Vitro* Fertilisation: Ethical and Legal Problems', presented at Women, Reproduction and Technology conference, 15 February.

Warnock, Mary (1987) 'The Limits of Toleration', The annual J. B. and W. B. Morrell Memorial Address on Toleration, University of York, 4 March.

Index

241